PRACTICAL PURSUITS

Takano Chōei, Takahashi

Keisaku, and Western Medicine in

Nineteenth-Century Japan

Harvard East Asian Monographs 255

PRACTICAL PURSUITS

Takano Chōei, Takahashi

Keisaku, and Western Medicine in

Nineteenth-Century Japan

Ellen Gardner Nakamura

Published by the Harvard University Asia Center
Distributed by Harvard University Press
Cambridge (Massachusetts) and London 2005

Printed in the United States of America

The Harvard University Asia Center publishes a monograph series and, in coordination with the Fairbank Center for East Asian Research, the Korea Institute, the Reischauer Institute of Japanese Studies, and other faculties and institutes, administers research projects designed to further scholarly understanding of China, Japan, Vietnam, Korea, and other Asian countries. The Center also sponsors projects addressing multidisciplinary and regional issues in Asia.

Library of Congress Cataloging-in-Publication Data

Nakamura, Ellen Gardner, 1971–

Practical pursuits : Takano Chōei, Takahashi Keisaku, and western medicine in nineteenth-century Japan / Ellen Gardner Nakamura.

p. cm.

Includes bibliographical references and index.

ISBN 0-674-01952-0 (cloth : alk. paper)

1. Takano, Chōei, 1804-1850. 2. Takahashi, Keisaku, 1799-1875. 3. Medicine--Japan--History--19th century. I. Title.

R624.N34 2005

610'.952--dc22

2005001938

Index by the author

❀ Printed on acid-free paper

Last figure below indicates year of this printing

15 14 13 12 11 10 09 08 07 06 05

Acknowledgments

I first came across the Japanese physician Takano Chōei (1804–50) as an undergraduate with a vague interest in the history of medicine. Even as a schoolchild, I vividly recall being gruesomely fascinated by reading about trephining: an ancient treatment that involved drilling a hole in the skull to allow bad spirits or a supernatural cause of disease to escape. During my teens, I became interested in herbs, acupuncture, and "alternative" medicines, and I even did a week of "work experience" surrounded by the heady smells of herbs and massage oils at the clinic of a local naturopath. Perhaps it was only natural, then, that when my studies eventually led me to the field of history, I should wish to write about medicine.

The discovery of the dramatic life story of Takano Chōei took me unexpectedly in another direction. Like many other historians before me, I found my attention initially directed to his political role, his imprisonment, and the place of Western scholarship in the modernization of Japan. As my work progressed, however, I gradually began to feel that there was more to his life and work than was generally told. Influenced by the work of Satō Shōsuke, I began to explore the idea that perhaps Chōei was much more a scholar and a physician than he was a political activist. My development of this line of thought was interrupted by another discovery.

During a period of study at Tokyo Gakugei University, I was introduced to a volume of Chōei's personal correspondence. These letters were a historian's delight; they ranged over a period from his earliest days as a youthful student in Edo through to his studies as a young man in Nagasaki and led right up to his escape from prison in 1844. The letters were long and rambling, written in a style that often said as much about its author as the content of the letters itself. I became fascinated not only by the picture they drew of Takano Chōei, the man, but also by the details I encountered of the way he trained and worked: the stuff of daily life.

Most of the letters in this collection were written to members of Chōei's family: his adoptive father, his uncle, and his cousin. Of the few remaining letters, one was addressed to Yanagida Teizō, a friend from the province of Kōzuke. Teizō was one of a number of doctors from this region who supported Chōei financially and helped with his works on famine relief and epidemic disease. I had been aware of the presence of these doctors for some time, from accounts in the work of Takano Chōun and Tsurumi Shunsuke. Principally, the doctors had been described in terms of the role they may have had in harboring Chōei after his escape from prison. Now I became interested in the Kōzuke physicians in their own right. How had Chōei come to develop such a geographically compact group of supporters? What made these doctors persevere with their country practices when Chōei had been so ruthlessly determined to lead an urban life? How did they go about their daily work? I learned that both Teizō and another member of the group, Takahashi Keisaku, had kept journals, and that these had been published (one quite recently). Luck was truly on my side, and gradually the outline of this study began to take shape.

So, with the writing of this book, my interest in Takano Chōei has finally brought me back to the history of medicine. This work has a social slant that I probably never would have dreamed of all those years ago when I found myself irresistibly attracted to the gory details of past medical practice, but my basic interest in the history of everyday life remains unchanged.

A great deal of my research time has necessarily been devoted to working my way slowly through the primary materials in a place and time far removed from that in which they were written. Nevertheless, like the rural doctors of my study, I have been supported by networks of friends and colleagues who have not allowed me to feel lonely or isolated for long. Throughout my PhD candidature at the Australian National University, I was blessed with conscientious and encouraging supervisors, supportive colleagues and administrators, and a comfortable working environment. At ANU, special thanks are due to my supervisors Tessa Morris-Suzuki, John Caiger, Anthea Hyslop, and Morris Low. Richard Mason provided helpful advice and endless encouragement. Colin Jeffcott and Bill Jenner kindly helped with the translation of sections from Chinese. Gavan McCormack and Iriye Takanori provided assistance in various ways. I am also grateful to the ANU's Cartographic Services at the Research School of Pacific and Asian Studies, and in particular to Kay Dancey, for the wonderful maps, and for permission to publish them in the book. In Japan, Takeuchi Makoto, Ōishi Manabu, Aoki Toshiyuki, Karasawa Sadaichi, Takahashi Tadao, and Ochiai Nobutaka all provided generous support. The staff at Kyoto University Library, in particular Ayabe Fusako, have been very helpful in providing illustrations. I am grateful to the library for permission to publish them. My colleagues at the University of Auckland, and in particular Richard Phillips, who generously read the entire manuscript and saved me from embarrassing errors, have been very supportive. Martha Chaiklin has been a friendly correspondent who has provided lots of help, especially with Dutch translations.

A shorter version of Chapter 3 first appeared as Ellen Gardner Nakamura, "Physicians and Famine in Japan: Takano Chōei in the 1830s," in *Social History of Medicine* 13, no. 3 (2000): 429–45, and is republished by kind permission of Oxford University Press. I would like to thank Ann Jannetta, an anonymous referee, and the editors of *Social History of Medicine* for their critical comments at that time. I am also deeply indebted to the two anonymous readers for the Harvard University Asia Center Publications Program for their helpful criticisms and advice and to Ann Klefstad for her prompt advice and editorial expertise. Any remaining errors are my own responsibility.

Finally, special thanks are due to my dear friends and family: to Yuko Asano, Bethwyn Evans, Rosemary Jeffcott, Buffy Ward, and

Karen Welberry for their warm companionship, both academic and otherwise, to my parents, Bernice and Colin, and in-laws Ryōzō and Fusako for their unfailing support, and most of all to Jun for not allowing me to give up.

E.G.N.

Contents

Maps and Figures

Maps

Figures

Notes to the Reader

Japanese names follow the convention of surname first, with the exception of writers publishing in English who follow the English word order. Please note, however, that after their first introduction, pre-Meiji historical figures are for the most part referred to using their first names or pseudonyms.

Macrons are supplied for long vowels except in cases where the word is common in the English language, such as "Tokyo." Other Japanese words that are commonly used in the field of Japanese studies have not been italicized, though they may bear macrons. Chinese words are romanized according to the Pinyin system.

Year dates have been converted to the Gregorian calendar. Names of months and days, however, have been left according to the lunar calendar and are rendered as in "the second day of the second month."

Unless otherwise indicated, all English translations of Japanese materials have been made by the author.

Tokugawa Currency

Three systems of currency operated in the Tokugawa period:

Gold currency
1 *ryō* = 4 *bu*
1 *bu* = 4 *shu*

Silver currency
1 *kanme* = 1,000 *monme*
1 *monme* = 10 *fun*

(Silver currency, cont.)
1 *fun* = 10 *rin*
1 *rin* = 10 *mō*

Copper currency
1 *kanmon* = 1,000 *mon*
10 *mon* = 1 *hiki*

Currency conversion rates fluctuated over time. In 1842, for example, the official rate was 1 gold *ryō* = 60 silver *monme* = 6,500 copper *mon*.

Meiji Currency

In 1868, silver currency was abolished, and the following year, one gold *ryō* was set at 10,000 copper *mon*. The yen was introduced in 1871 and was equivalent to two gold *bu* of Tokugawa currency. Meiji currency worked according to a decimal system:

1 (gold) yen = 100 (copper) *sen*
1 *sen* = 10 *rin*

Tokugawa Weights and Measures

1 *sun* = 1.2 inches (3.03 cm)
10 *sun* = 1 *shaku* = 0.994 foot (30.3 cm)
1 *shaku* = 0.0384 pint (0.018 liter)
10 *shaku* = 1 *gō* = 0.384 pint (0.18 liter)
10 *gō* = 1 *shō* = 1.92 quarts (1.8 liters)
1 *rin* = 0.001325 ounce (0.0375 grams)
10 *rin* = 1 *fun* = 0.01325 ounce (0.375 grams)
10 *fun* = 1 *monme* = 0.1325 ounce (3.75 grams)

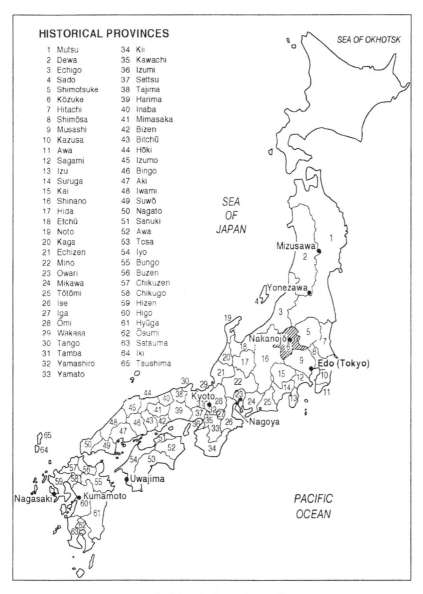

HISTORICAL PROVINCES

1	Mutsu	34	Kii
2	Dewa	35	Kawachi
3	Echigo	36	Izumi
4	Sado	37	Settsu
5	Shimotsuke	38	Tajima
6	Kōzuke	39	Harima
7	Hitachi	40	Inaba
8	Shimōsa	41	Mimasaka
9	Musashi	42	Bizen
10	Kazusa	43	Bitchū
11	Awa	44	Hōki
12	Sagami	45	Izumo
13	Izu	46	Bingo
14	Suruga	47	Aki
15	Kai	48	Iwami
16	Shinano	49	Suwō
17	Hida	50	Nagato
18	Etchū	51	Sanuki
19	Noto	52	Awa
20	Kaga	53	Tosa
21	Echizen	54	Iyo
22	Mino	55	Bungo
23	Owari	56	Buzen
24	Mikawa	57	Chikuzen
25	Tōtōmi	58	Chikugo
26	Ise	59	Hizen
27	Iga	60	Higo
28	Ōmi	61	Hyūga
29	Wakasa	62	Ōsumi
30	Tango	63	Satsuma
31	Tamba	64	Iki
32	Yamashiro	65	Tsushima
33	Yamato		

SEA OF OKHOTSK

SEA OF JAPAN

Mizusawa

Yonezawa

Nakanojō

Edo (Tokyo)

Kyoto

Nagoya

Uwajima

Nagasaki

Kumamoto

PACIFIC OCEAN

Map 1   The historical provinces of Japan.
Courtesy of Cartographic Services, Research School of Pacific and
Asian Studies, The Australian National University.

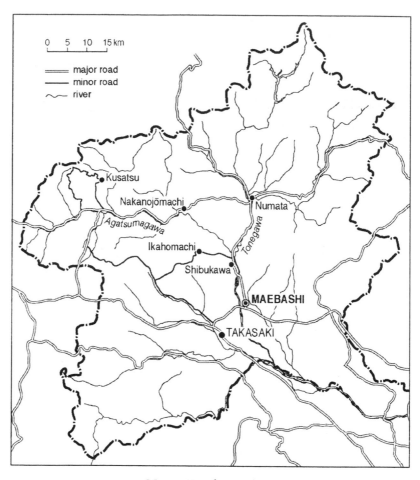

Map 2 Kōzuke province.
Courtesy of Cartographic Services, Research School of Pacific
and Asian Studies, The Australian National University.

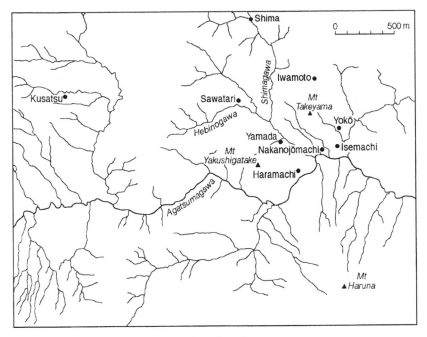

Map 3   The Nakanojō region.
Courtesy of Cartographic Services, Research School of Pacific
and Asian Studies, The Australian National University.

PRACTICAL PURSUITS

Takano Chōei, Takahashi

Keisaku, and Western Medicine in

Nineteenth-Century Japan

Introduction

The history of Western medicine in the late Tokugawa period is usually depicted as a prelude to modern medicine.[1] By comparison to the Western medical science that was systematically introduced in the Meiji period, the Tokugawa study of Western learning is often seen as a hopelessly backward exercise in which inadequately equipped Japanese doctors valiantly struggled to make sense of outdated Dutch knowledge. In contrast, I argue here that the study of Western medicine was actually a dynamic activity that brought together doctors from all over the country in efforts to effect social change. Western knowledge was not simply the property of elite samurai doctors working for the Bakufu or domains but was shared even by commoner doctors working in local practice in rural backwaters.[2] Through the examples of the doctors Takano Chōei (1804-50) and Takahashi Keisaku (1799-1875), this book explores the context into which local Japanese doctors incorporated Western ideas, the social networks through which they communicated them, and the geographical spaces that supported these activities. By examining the social impact of Western learning at the level of everyday life, rather than simply its impact at the theoreti-

---

1. On the pitfalls of writing premodern history, see Gluck, "The Invention of Edo."

2. The Tokugawa status system recognized four classes: samurai (warriors), farmers, artisans, and merchants. There were also various groups of people who suffered discrimination and were considered to be outside this system. "Commoner" in this book refers to anyone who was not a samurai or a member of an "outcaste" group.

cal level, the book offers a broad picture of the way in which Western medicine was absorbed and adapted in Japan.

The two case studies provide something of a contrast. Takano Chōei was one of the most talented scholars of Western learning in nineteenth-century Japan, although, as we shall see, he never quite reached his full potential, either socially or academically. Hailing originally from the countryside in northern Honshu, he became an ambitious urban man who was a scholar first and a doctor second. Takahashi Keisaku, on the other hand, was simply a rural doctor from the province of Kōzuke (present-day Gunma, in the northwest Kanto region). He lived most of his life in obscurity in the countryside. It is he who provides the most powerful example of the permeation of Western knowledge into remote corners of Japan.

The approach taken in this book ties in with a burgeoning field of history in Japan: *zaison no rangaku,* or "study of Western learning in the countryside." For a long time in Japanese historiography, the study of Western knowledge was regarded as something belonging to the warrior class. This interpretation came about because of a focus on the history of the ruling elites, of great men, and on intellectual and technological history rather than social history.[3] In particular, after the events of the *bansha no goku* in 1839, in which Western learning was severely repressed (see below), many historians thought that Western knowledge was more or less incorporated into the mechanisms of the Bakufu government, to be used for the rulers' own purposes. Yet, as isolated local studies can now demonstrate, Western learning was alive and well in the countryside, in the hands of members of the rural elite.

The introduction of Western learning was a creative and adaptive process. Whereas one scholar in his intellectual history could only conclude that Western learning in Japan was "a kind of miscellaneous collection of practical data and techniques without cohesive structure or inner meaning" and that the central role played by physicians actually curbed rather than promoted the possibility of critical thought,[4] I argue that Western learning did indeed have a

---

3. See Aoki Toshiyuki's historiographical discussion in *Zaison rangaku no kenkyū,* pp. 3–8.

4. Goodman, *Japan: The Dutch Experience,* pp. 228–30.

meaning in Japan. My aim is not to dispute the unsystematic manner in which Western knowledge was appropriated; rather, I question the terms on which it has been historically evaluated.

From the start, Western learning in Japan was closely associated with practical and social problems. As Tetsuo Najita has put it, "Dutch was a language to translate, not to theorize with."[5] The study of Western knowledge was not frivolous, despite the development of a popular form.[6] Takano Chōei wrote that "the reason why we *rangaku* scholars study Western learning against all odds is because it is rational and taking it as one's calling is useful."[7] Western learning was thus justified in terms of *jitsugaku,* or "practical learning." This term became popular during the early modern period in Japan among Confucianists, statesmen, philosophers, *rangaku* scholars, and patriots. Sometimes practical learning is interpreted as a progressive strand of thought that arose in opposition to traditional Neo-Confucian thought. Yet the term *jitsugaku* originated within Neo-Confucianism itself, as a contrast to the "empty learning" of Buddhism and Taoism. Many types of rational, empirical, and practical learning originated within Neo-Confucian thought, and as time passed, *jitsugaku* came to be identified with various values or activities within the Confucian framework that dealt with the practical needs of society. Some of these values were "moral solidity," "social applicability," and "intellectual substantiality."[8] Concepts such as these could easily be used to justify the study of Western knowledge, especially when the subject matter had a practical application, such as famine relief. It therefore seems appropriate to examine the serious study of Western learning in the same practical and social terms in which it was taken up, rather than simply in terms of a trajectory of modernization.

---

5. Najita, "History and Nature in Eighteenth-Century Tokugawa Thought," p. 634.

6. The popularization of Western knowledge in Japan (particularly its application to "nonfunctional uses") is explored in Screech, *The Western Scientific Gaze.*

7. Takano Chōei, "Wasuregatami," p. 182. An alternative title for this work is *Tori no naku ne* (The cry of a bird).

8. Wm. Theodore de Bary, "Introduction," in *Principle and Practicality,* p. 32.

The Development of *Rangaku*

The story of the introduction of Western knowledge to Japan during the Edo period (1603–1868) has often been told. It is usually the tale of a small group of Japanese men who, against all odds, battled to learn the Dutch language and something of the world from which they had been "isolated." The exchange between these men and the isolated European physicians who taught them (who lived on the tiny artificial island of Dejima, off the trading post of Nagasaki) took place despite the limitations of a foreign policy that restricted international contact for approximately two hundred years, and it has captured the imagination of historians in Japan and the West alike.

In fact, the nature of the maritime restrictions (*kaikin*) enforced by the Tokugawa government has been the source of many misconceptions in both Japanese and Western scholarship. This stems partly from the popularity of the term "closed country" (*sakoku*) to refer to the Japan of this period, though in fact this was a misleading term coined by a European visitor, which only later came into use.[9] The maritime restrictions were more about controlling foreign relations than cutting them off; they were in part an effort to rid Japan of Catholicism and to control trade. Implemented gradually from 1633–39 and continuing until 1853, they placed strict limitations on travel abroad and on foreign ships wishing to enter Japan.

The Tokugawa government attempted to control official foreign trade by permitting it only at the port of Nagasaki, and only with selected trading partners. However, it also authorized certain domains such as Satsuma and Tsushima to trade with China, the Ryūkyū Islands, Korea, and the Ainu people of Ezo (Hokkaido). Trade, particularly with Asia, was therefore a vital part of Tokugawa foreign policy. The emphasis in history writing on the Tokugawa state's isolation has come partly through a preoccupation with Japan's relations with Western nations. Holland was the only

---

9. The word *sakoku* was not used in Japan until the nineteenth century, when the Nagasaki scholar Shitsuki Tadao translated the Dutch version of Engelbert Kaempfer's (1651–1716) *The History of Japan* into Japanese in 1801. See Toby, *State and Diplomacy in Early Modern Japan*, pp. 12–13.

Western nation to be granted permission to continue trading with the Japanese after the implementation of the maritime prohibitions. Since England had already withdrawn from the scene because it found the trade unprofitable, the main country to be affected by the laws in their initial stages was Portugal. While the Portuguese had made themselves unpopular through their zealous Catholic missionary activity, the Dutch on the other hand had prudently demonstrated that they were interested only in trade. They even went so far as to come to the military aid of the Tokugawa government when it put down an uprising of poor Christian peasants at Shimabara on the island of Kyushu in 1638.[10]

As Ronald Toby has convincingly demonstrated, however, ridding the country of Christianity was not the only dimension to this policy of maritime restrictions. In the 1630s, the Tokugawa government was still relatively new. Under the leadership of Tokugawa Ieyasu, the Tokugawa family had in 1600 emerged victorious from a battle to reunify the country after a long period of civil war. The system of government developed by Ieyasu was a federation of around 260 domains (*han*). These domains were ruled by autonomous lords called "daimyo," who retained their autonomy on the condition that they swore fealty to the Tokugawa military government, known as the Bakufu. It was therefore very important to the fledgling Bakufu government to strengthen the position of the Tokugawa family over the other daimyo lords. For this reason, daimyo were not permitted to engage in foreign trade or to build ships over a certain size. Furthermore, the policy was designed to give Japan, and the Tokugawa government in particular, a new sense of identity within the Asian region. By controlling foreign relations, the Tokugawa could place themselves firmly at the center of the universe.[11]

Because of its special role in the conduct of official foreign trade, the port of Nagasaki came to be a center for Western learning in

---

10. On the Shimabara Rebellion, see Morris, *The Nobility of Failure*, pp. 143–79.
11. See Keene, *The Japanese Discovery of Europe*, pp. 1–2; Wakabayashi, *Anti-Foreignism and Western Learning in Early Modern Japan*, p. 61; and Toby, *State and Diplomacy in Early Modern Japan*, especially pp. 211–30.

Japan.[12] It was through Nagasaki that Western goods and books were imported, and it was on the manmade island of Dejima just off the coast that the Dutch traders were required to live. The traders had only limited contact with Japanese people, and they conducted their business through official interpreters who were assigned to them. By all accounts, the skills of these translators were fairly rudimentary, and initially they worked in Portuguese rather than Dutch, but they nevertheless formed a starting point for the scholastic endeavor that eventually came to be known as *rangaku*.[13]

Although the word *rangaku* literally means "Dutch learning," the books studied in Japan included not only Dutch books but Chinese translations of them, in addition to Dutch translations of other European works. Therefore, the word *rangaku* should be understood broadly to refer to European knowledge, particularly concerning medicine and technology, which was obtained through the medium of books imported at Nagasaki during the Edo period. Eventually, in the late nineteenth century, the term *yōgaku*, or "Western learning," came to replace the word *rangaku* because it more accurately reflected the fact that Holland was not the only subject of inquiry. In all other respects, the terms may be thought of as synonymous.[14]

Early interpreters tended to concentrate on basic oral communication. They passed on their skills from father to son, and their occupations became hereditary. Theirs was a serious business: they received their stipends from the Nagasaki governor and were made to promise to conduct trade in a proper manner, to report any religious activities they should encounter, and not to accept any presents.[15]

This was typical of the cautious approach to Western knowledge in the early Tokugawa period. Apart from the linguistic difficulties involved in reading Dutch works, the study of Western knowledge in Japan was fraught with difficulty for ideological rea-

---

12. It was also because of this special role that the governance of Nagasaki remained under the direct control of the Bakufu.

13. Numata, *Yōgaku*, p. 20.

14. Ibid., p. 1.

15. Ibid., p. 12.

sons as well. Due to the contemporary ban on Christianity and a fear among official circles that Western knowledge could lead to the moral subversion of the populace, the importation of Western books, particularly those in Chinese translation, was strictly controlled. Nevertheless, even in the early seventeenth century, daimyo were sending students to Nagasaki to learn from the doctors and translators there. Despite their imperfect skills, the information that they obtained was carefully shrouded in secrecy and monopolized by the Bakufu government and daimyo elites.[16]

Gradually, especially under the encouraging policies of the eighth shogun, Tokugawa Yoshimune (ruled 1716–45), *rangaku* began to develop into a field of scholarship.[17] In 1720, Yoshimune allowed the importation of certain Chinese astronomical and mathematical texts that had previously been banned because they had been written by, or reflected the ideas of, Christian missionaries in China.[18] In addition to the study of Dutch language, calendrical studies, and other practical subjects, Yoshimune also encouraged the cultivation of medicinal herbs and the promotion of public health policies to deal with epidemic disease.[19] Equally important to Yoshimune's patronage, however, was the general background of economic development and a growing interest in natural science.[20] From this time, there was a gradual change in the way that *rangaku* was perceived. Rather than being seen as a threat, Western learning was recognized as having practical benefits, particularly in relation to the scientific and technological needs that were arising from commercial developments.[21]

Furthermore, along with the relaxation of policy toward *rangaku* in the eighteenth century came a more general popularization of foreign things. This was the age of *ranpeki*, or "Dutch-crazy" people, who were fascinated by all kinds of Western objects and art. Unlike the serious *rangaku* scholars, those addicted to the craze

---

16. Ibid., pp. 31–36.
17. See Sippel, "Aoki Konyō (1698–1769) and the Beginnings of *Rangaku*."
18. Ibid., p. 128.
19. Ōishi, *Yoshimune to Kyōhō no kaikaku*, pp. 162–83.
20. Satō, *Yōgakushi kenkyū josetsu*, p. 79.
21. Numata, *Yōgaku*, pp. 72–74.

were more likely to be searching for "exotica" and "thrills" than anything else, and only the wealthiest could afford to collect Dutch objects themselves. Even so, those of lesser means were not immune and flocked to see foreign things in sideshows or to look at pictures in books.[22] Some rich daimyo and merchants contributed to serious intellectual pursuits by becoming patrons of *rangaku* scholars.[23]

By the late eighteenth century, thanks to improvements in linguistic skills among the interpreters and a supportive social and political environment, written Dutch materials were being sought as a source of scholarly knowledge. From the outset, much of the knowledge obtained through *rangaku* scholarship had been medical. This situation developed partly because of the activities of a succession of European doctors who came to Dejima to care for the health of the Europeans who lived there. Several of the doctors also attempted to learn as much as they could about Japan's natural history and culture, and the contributions of men such as Engelbert Kaempfer (1651–1716) and Philipp Franz von Siebold (1796–1866) to European knowledge of Japan are well known. The doctors also passed on some of their medical techniques to their official interpreters, some of whom later went into medical practice themselves.[24] Furthermore, medicine was better tolerated than many other fields of Western scholarship within the conservative climate of Tokugawa society because of its tangible practical benefits.

The beginning of scholarly *rangaku* is sometimes pinpointed as the publication of *Kaitai shinsho* (New treatise on dissection) in 1774.[25] This groundbreaking work did much to fuel the growing interest in Dutch learning and was especially important for the development of medicine. When Sugita Genpaku (1733–1817) and Maeno Ryōtaku (1723–1803) attended a dissection in 1771 and compared what they saw there with diagrams of the human body in Johann Adam Kulmus's *Tafel anatomia* (1731), they found them to

---

22. For a comprehensive examination of this topic, see Screech, *The Western Scientific Gaze.*
23. Numata, *Yōgaku*, pp. 77–78.
24. Ogawa, *Igaku no rekishi*, pp. 99–100.
25. Numata, *Yōgaku*, p. 96.

be remarkably accurate, while the traditional Chinese ones they had known up until then were grossly simplified. This inspired them to make a translation of the book, which they eventually published, with official sanction, as *Kaitai shinsho* in 1774.[26] The work of Genpaku and his colleagues was important because their conclusions were based on empirical observation rather than the speculative theories of Confucian medicine. Although their dissection was not the first to be conducted in Japan, it was the first to employ a new "way of seeing," in which the participants were not simply content to confirm the old theories, but were open to the new perceptions that Kulmus's anatomical work offered them.[27]

The model of medicine that Genpaku eventually proposed, based on an understanding of anatomy, did not become the norm until the Meiji period. Nevertheless, the work of the Western anatomists caused something of a crisis in Japanese medicine at the time. It was gradually recognized that Confucian medical theories were incompatible with the objective observation of reality.[28] This resonated with other developments in Confucian scholarship during the eighteenth century that began to question the status quo, and in particular with scholars who focused on the study of nature as the ultimate object of scholarly enquiry.[29]

Genpaku became one of the founders of a school of medicine known as *ranpō*, or "Dutch style" medicine, as opposed to *kanpō*, "Chinese style." The *ranpō* doctors studied and translated Dutch medical texts, and were particularly interested in anatomy and surgery. In practical terms, the medicine that they practiced was Western medicine in name, not necessarily in nature, as *ranpō* was still very much a blend of Chinese and Western methods. Nevertheless, it is equally important to recognize that in theoretical terms, they had divorced themselves from the Confucian framework of Chinese medicine. This development should not be seen as theirs alone, but within the context of other changes within Chinese medicine.

---

26. Keene, *The Japanese Discovery*, pp. 20–24.
27. Kuriyama, "Between Mind and Eye," p. 27.
28. Johnston, "Jūhasseiki Nihon no igaku ni okeru kagaku kakumei."
29. Najita, "History and Nature in Eighteenth-Century Tokugawa Thought."

Apart from *ranpō* medicine, five other schools of medicine can be identified in Tokugawa Japan. Most of these were grounded in Chinese medical thought, which had been brought to Japan by Korean doctors as early as the fifth century.[30] According to this Confucian view of the world, the human body was a microcosm of the macrocosmic universe and was thus subject to the same rules. The universe operated according to a complex system that was influenced by factors such as the "five evolutionary phases"; yin and yang; types of energy such as *qi* (*ki* in Japanese); and a numerical system based on the sexagenary cycle. The "five evolutionary phases" were earth, water, fire, metal, and wood, which interacted according to relationships of mutual productivity and conquest. All phenomena, starting with the five organs of the body, could be classified according to these elements. For example, the liver, the color blue, the planet Jupiter, the feeling of anger, and so on belonged to the wood element. The interactions of the "evolutionary phases" affected the state of balance within the body, and when the balance was upset through climatic, moral, nutritional, emotional, or other reasons, ill health was the result. Medical practitioners therefore required a thorough understanding of Confucian thought, though as Margaret Lock has pointed out, the system was also flexible enough to accommodate the rise of many different schools.[31]

By the Edo period, Japanese versions of Chinese medicine had developed to varying degrees into something quite different from Chinese medical theories, though they were based on Chinese medicine. The most fundamental change (though it did not occur in every school) was a move toward an understanding of medicine based on empirical evidence rather than on Confucian philosophy. Prior to Genpaku's *Kaitai shinsho*, some schools conducted autopsies and anatomical experiments despite the traditional taboo on dissection, and it has been argued that they gradually paved the way for the acceptance of Western medicine in Japan.[32]

---

30. Ogawa, *Igaku no rekishi*, p. 30.
31. Lock, *East Asian Medicine in Urban Japan*, p. 48.
32. See Johnston, "Jūhasseiki Nihon no igaku ni okeru kagaku kakumei."

The most important school in the early Edo period was the *go-seiha* ("latter-day") or *rishu* school. It developed in Japan in the sixteenth century and was influenced by Chinese medicine of the Jin and Yuan periods (ca. 1125–1368). As a school of thought, it was based on Neo-Confucian metaphysical principles, and its texts were highly theoretical. On the other hand, it also had a more practical side, and some of the speculative elements of the theory had been removed.[33] *Rishu* doctors advocated a holistic approach to the body and the achievement of bodily balance through the administration of gentle medicines.[34] This school was represented by Tashiro Sanki (1465–1537), who had studied in China, and his pupil Manase Dōsan (1507–94), of Kyoto. It flourished until the beginning of the eighteenth century.

The *goseiha* school was eclipsed around this time by the *koihō* ("old way of medicine") school, popularized by Gotō Konzan (1659–1733) and Yoshimasu Tōdō (1702–73). The development of the *koihō* school of Chinese medicine paralleled the rise of *kogaku* (classical studies) in Confucian scholarship. Both movements called for a return to Chinese classics. In particular, the *koihō* scholars rejected the speculative ideas of *rishu* medicine and advocated a return to a book called the *Shang han lun* (*Shōkanron* in Japanese), which was written around AD 200 and was predominantly a practical textbook of pharmacotherapeutics.[35] Eventually *koihō* medicine split into two streams: one centered on Tōdō's clinical experimentation, and one developed by Yamawaki Tōyō (1705–62), who stressed the importance of basic medicine. In particular, Tōyō and his followers divorced themselves from Confucian thought to create a new anatomical understanding of the body, and dissection was an important part of their work.[36]

The *kōshōgaku* ("historical investigation") school was led by the Taki family, one of the most powerful medical families in the Edo period. Taki Genkō (1695–1766) had a formidable pedigree; he was a descendant of Tanba Yasuyori (912–95), author of *Ishinpō*, the

---

33. Ibid., p. 10.
34. Lock, *East Asian Medicine in Urban Japan*, p. 53.
35. Otsuka, "Chinese Traditional Medicine in Japan," pp. 323–25.
36. Johnston, "Jūhasseiki Nihon no igaku ni okeru kagaku kakumei," p. 15.

oldest extant medical book in Japan. Taki Genkō was made an official Bakufu doctor in 1747, and the private school that he had founded, the Seijukan, became the Bakufu's official medical school in 1791. Thereafter, the Taki family were its hereditary directors.[37] While continuing its function as a training center, the school also had responsibility for official publications.[38] The Taki family and their followers emphasized a minute examination of Chinese and Japanese medical classics and were influenced by a similar movement in Confucian studies. The group made a great contribution to classical studies, but remained steadfastly conservative in its medical approach.[39]

Toward the end of the Edo period, another group of doctors, known as the *wahō* ("Japanese way") school, tried to find a uniquely "Japanese" way of healing by studying the Japanese classics. They were obviously influenced by the then-new national learning (*kokugaku*) movement. Motoori Norinaga (1730–1801), founder of the movement, was by profession a provincial doctor. He emphasized observation based on the five senses and experience, rather than the theoretical constructs of Chinese medicine. He believed that on an everyday level, Chinese medicine had become naturalized, and he was not troubled by the fact that the medicine he practiced was Chinese in origin.[40] Ueda Akinari (1734–1809) and Tanigawa Kotosuga (1709–76), also doctor-scholars, were similar in this respect. Later, Hirata Atsutane (1776–1843) argued that all medicine (including Chinese and Dutch) was given to the world by the two gods, Ōanamuchi-no-kami and Sukuna-biko-na-no-kami. In 1852, a doctor and *kokugaku* scholar from Sunpu called Hananoi Yūnen wrote *Ihō seiden* (A true account of medicine), in which, like Atsutane, he argued that Japanese gods had given medicine to the world, but that foreign countries had lost this information.[41] He claimed there was a need to test the wisdom of Chinese knowledge on Japanese soil, because diseases and medicines differed from

---

37. Hattori, *Edo jidai igakushi no kenkyū*, p. 13.
38. Ogawa, *Igaku no rekishi*, pp. 154–55.
39. Hattori, *Edo jidai igakushi no kenkyū*, pp. 13–14.
40. Ibid., p. 152.
41. Ibid., p. 154. Tsukamoto gives the date for this work as 1851.

country to country. Thus, he emphasized practical, traditional knowledge, rather than (Chinese) written knowledge. He asserted that disease came from abroad and that Japan was a land without indigenous diseases. Illnesses that were not brought to Japan by foreigners were caused when the gods went on a rampage.[42]

The *kanransetchū* ("Chinese-Dutch eclectic") school was in some respects an extension of the developments in *koihō* medicine. Indeed, Yamawaki Tōyō is sometimes considered to belong to this school. These doctors engaged in experimental work and were influenced by the study of Western anatomy. They began to introduce elements of Western medicine into their practice, particularly in the areas of surgery, bloodletting, and obstetrics.[43] Hanaoka Seishū (1760–1835), who is representative of this school, saw a need to unify surgery and internal medicine. He became famous for his innovations in surgery. In particular, he was remarkable for his development and use of an anesthetic in 1805, forty years before it was developed in the West. The medicine consisted of a mixture of six crude drugs from the traditional Chinese pharmacopoeia.[44] It included both aconite and datura, which were noted for their anesthetizing, and poisonous, qualities. In the process of refining the drug, Seishū used his wife Kae as a human subject, an experiment that caused her to lose her sight.[45] The story of her sacrifice has been fictionalized by Ariyoshi Sawako in a novel that explores the traditional relationships between man, wife, and mother.[46]

Thus, in terms of medical thought, the latter half of the Edo period was a time of great intellectual debate, much as it was for Confucian scholarship in general. There were certainly conservative Chinese doctors who resolutely clung to the old speculative theories. Yet there were other doctors of Chinese medicine who were looking for new answers. Western medicine was incorporated as one part of this exciting intellectual scene.

---

42. Tsukamoto, *Tokai to inaka*, pp. 239–42.
43. Fujikawa, *Nihon igakushi kōyō*, 2: 11–13.
44. Kodansha, ed., *Kodansha Encyclopedia of Japan*, 3: 94.
45. Nichiran Gakkai, ed., *Yōgakushi jiten*, p. 573.
46. Ariyoshi, *The Doctor's Wife*.

Historiography

The history of Western medicine in Japan, as an important part of *rangaku* scholarship, has often been treated in both Western and Japanese scholarship as a straightforward account of the lives of important men, their discoveries, and the march toward the attainment of modern medicine and "progress."[47] Heroes such as Sugita Genpaku often figure prominently in such accounts. On the other hand, this approach has led in some cases to a culturally blinkered perspective. Some works have treated the history of medicine in Japan during the Tokugawa and Meiji periods by detailing the experiences and successes of the series of Western physicians at Nagasaki, paying only scant attention to the Japanese who worked with them.[48] Another Western scholar demonstrated his Eurocentric approach by berating the early modern Japanese for taking on board only Western technology without Western ideology.[49] Even in cases where an author was basically free from such biases, often the aim was still to chart a history of conceptual "progress" from Chinese to Western medicine.[50] More recently, however, Dutch scholars have undertaken some interesting work on the history of medicine that differs from this. One writer, for example, turned the traditional Dutch-Japanese relationship on its head by writing about the introduction of acupuncture to the West.[51]

---

47. See, for example, Hattori, *Edo jidai igakushi no kenkyū*, or, more recently, Koike, *Zusetsu Nihon no 'i' no rekishi*. An exception is the following innovative collection of essays on a wide range of medical topics: Kuriyama and Yamada, eds., *Rekishi no naka no yamai to igaku*.

48. See Bowers, *Western Medical Pioneers in Feudal Japan*; and idem, *When the Twain Meet*. The emphasis chosen by Bowers may in part be explained by the fact that his work is largely based on materials held in European archives, and his bibliography contains few Japanese sources.

49. Goodman, *Japan: The Dutch Experience*, p. 228. Using an impressive collection of Japanese works, Goodman alleges the "valuelessness" of *rangaku*, for this reason.

50. See Ozaki, "Conceptual Changes in Japanese Medicine During the Tokugawa Period."

51. Haneveld, "The Introduction of Acupuncture into Western Medicine: The Influence of Japanese and Dutch Physicians."

Early Japanese scholarship, too, tended to focus on biographical, bibliographical, and technological histories of Western learning in Japan.[52] As more general histories came to be written, they attempted, under the influence of Marxist scholarship, to define the role of Western knowledge in the process of modernization. Scholars searching for the historical significance of *rangaku* typically were divided into two schools: those who believed that *rangaku* had a role in reinforcing the feudal system and ideology and those who believed that proponents of *rangaku* were opposed to the feudal system and helped to overthrow it.[53]

Scholars such as Itō Tasaburō (1909–84), who argued that *rangaku* scholarship reinforced the feudal system, claimed that, although Western learning was progressive, this did not necessarily mean that it overcame feudalism, and that the "self-restrictive character of *Rangaku* served . . . as a prop to feudal society."[54] In other words, these scholars emphasized the way in which the Tokugawa regime harnessed scholars of Western learning and used them to its own advantage, thereby hampering "progress." On the other hand, Marxist scholars such as Hani Goro (1901–83) and Takahashi Shinichi (1913–85) suggested that there was an anti-feudal, progressive element to Western learning in Japan.[55] Tōyama Shigeki (1914–) argued that a repression like that of 1839 could only mean that some kind of revolution against the old way of thinking had occurred. This revolution was effectively suppressed, however, by the Bakufu government, with the result that *rangaku* scholars thereafter channeled their efforts into policies for strengthening the country and army.[56]

Numata Jirō's (1912–94) early work was an extension of that of Itō Tasaburō. His later research was quite broad-ranging, but it also tended to focus on the protective role that the Bakufu played with regard to *rangaku* scholarship. For Numata, *rangaku* devel-

---

52. For a more comprehensive review of the writing of *rangaku* history, see Numata, "Studies of the History of Yōgaku."

53. Satō, *Yōgakushi kenkyū josetsu*, p. 4.

54. Numata, "Studies of the History of Yōgaku."

55. Ibid.

56. Satō, *Yōgakushi kenkyū josetsu*, pp. 4–7.

oped out of very practical and political needs associated with up-
holding a policy of resistance toward Western nations, and it was
this aspect that ultimately rendered it insufficient when faced with
the systematic modern knowledge that was imported in the Meiji
period.[57] He even saw the Bakufu's response to the Siebold Affair
and the events of 1839 as rather restrained, and noted how the officials quickly moved to re-monopolize Western learning, rather
than to try to stamp it out.[58] Numata did, however, recognize the
importance of personal contact in the introduction of Western
knowledge and called for further work in the area of private studies and regional histories.[59]

One further Japanese historian worthy of mention here is Satō
Shōsuke (1918–97). Satō placed importance on the development of
Confucian *kogaku* thought as a foundation for the systematic introduction of Western science. In this, he disagreed fundamentally
with Numata, who believed that until the end of the Tokugawa
period, *rangaku* was only ever a haphazard accumulation of practical knowledge. While the two scholars appear to have had quite a
fiery professional relationship, perhaps their differences are not ir-
reconcilable. Satō appears to have been mostly searching for the
roots of *rangaku* scholarship, and he found these in the changes in
Confucian scholarship associated with *kogaku*.[60] Numata, on the
other hand, seems to have been looking back from the perspective
of the gap between *rangaku* (or *yōgaku*) and modern Western
medicine at the beginning of the Meiji period. He noted the practical and unsystematic nature of *rangaku*, arguing that most of it had
little to do with Confucian philosophy. Certainly the changes in
Chinese medicine inspired by *kogaku* scholarship appear to have
prepared the way for the interest in Western medicine, as outlined
above. Numata is right, however, to emphasize the practicality of
rangaku scholarship thereafter and its differences from modern science. There is something to be learned from both points of view.

---

57. Numata, *Yōgaku*, pp. 234–45.
58. Ibid., p. 242.
59. Numata, "Studies of the History of Yōgaku."
60. Satō, *Yōgakushi kenkyū josetsu*, pt. I.

Takano Chōei

The politicization of *rangaku* in history writing is nowhere more obvious than in the treatment of Takano Chōei, one of its most famous scholars. Despite the fact that he wrote many medical works and was a prolific translator, Chōei is mostly remembered as a political figure. In some ways, this is hardly surprising. Along with Watanabe Kazan (1793–1841) and Koseki San'ei (1787–1839), Chōei was a victim of what has become known as the *bansha no goku*: literally, the "imprisonment of barbarian associates." This was a dramatic repression of Western studies by the Bakufu government in 1839, and it had far-reaching repercussions for *rangaku* scholarship. In many works of history, this episode has been portrayed as a battle between old and new knowledge. The repression is blamed on the culmination of fierce jealousies and fears within the powerful Confucian establishment that its official doctrine would be undermined.

Chōei's crime was to have authored *Bojutsu yume monogatari* (The tale of a dream), an essay criticizing the application of the "shell and repel" edict on foreign ships.[61] This edict was promulgated in 1825 and ordered that foreign ships invading Japanese waters be sent away immediately and by violent means if necessary, without providing provisions or other assistance.[62] Chōei was prompted to write the tale in response to news he heard about the hostile treatment of the American ship *Morrison*, which had approached Uraga Bay in 1837. He argued that this was a dangerous policy that could insult the foreigners and turn them against the Japanese. In fact, Chōei's understanding of this event was rather flawed. He had not learned of the arrival of the *Morrison* until nearly a year after the event, and moreover, he mistook the name of the ship for a well-known English missionary in China, Dr. Robert Morrison (1782–1834), who had actually died prior to

---

61. *Bojutsu* referred to the year in which it was written: 1838.

62. Although the edict has often been interpreted as an example of Japan's xenophobic policies, at the time it was conceived of largely as an attempt to control unruly foreign whaling ships. See Steele and Caiger, "On Ignorant Whalers and Japan's 'Shell and Repel' Edict of 1825."

the ship's arrival. Chōei argued that to treat an eminent person such as Morrison with such disrespect would arouse hostility among the Europeans.[63]

In many accounts of Chōei's life, he has been glorified as a man who was tragically imprisoned, and eventually died, for his role in the modernization of his country. Sadly, however, this has meant that these political events have been allowed to overshadow the significance of his early career, and the medical work on which his reputation was built has been rather neglected.

Scholarly work on Chōei first became popular in the Meiji period (1868–1912). One of the first and most influential studies was a book entitled *Bunmei tōzenshi* (A history of civilization's eastward advance), published in 1884 by Fujita Mokichi (1852–92). Fujita, who was a graduate of Fukuzawa Yukichi's Keio Gijuku and a participant in the civil liberties movement, tended to see Chōei and Kazan as forefathers of that movement and to glorify them as martyrs to the feudal system.[64] His work provided the basis for many popular ideas about Chōei, both in the Meiji period and beyond.

In 1898, Chōei received a posthumous official pardon from the Meiji Emperor, and a commemorative stone was erected the following year. These events seem to have inspired further research on his life, for there was something of a Chōei boom over the next decade. According to one bibliography, there were six books and one article published between 1898, the year of his pardon, and 1913.[65]

The most significant of the writers of this period was Takano Chōun (1862–1946). Chōun was a descendant of the Takano family (though he was not a blood relation of Chōei) and he too was a doctor. He published the first edition of his important work *Takano Chōei den*, a biography of Chōei, in 1928. A second edition was published in 1943. In the preface to this edition, he explained the reasons behind his efforts:

I began the study of my ancestor Chōei fifty-two years ago, in the twenty-third year of Meiji (1890). . . . As Chōei was a wanted criminal,

63. See Takano Chōei, "Wasuregatami."
64. Satō, *Yōgakushi kenkyū josetsu*, pp. 131–33.
65. Nichiran Gakkai, ed., *Yōgaku kankei kenkyū bunken yōran*.

many of those who had been connected to him had purposely burned their documents in order to hide the truth. Fifty years after his death, his friends and acquaintances had already died, and evidence had disappeared without trace into oblivion, so my investigations were fraught with difficulty. . . . Even after his death, it is regrettable that, for many years, novelistic biographies of Chōei continued to propagate mistakes. I thought, as his descendant, it was my duty to publish a true biography and correct all the false accounts. For this reason, I resolved that no matter how difficult, or what sacrifices I might have to make, I would not stop until I collapsed, and earnestly went about collecting materials.[66]

Chōun's biography was thus something of a personal quest, and its eulogistic nature must be taken into account when reading it. It nevertheless contains many documents and letters, and it remains a detailed and useful account. Chōun followed up the biography with the publication of four volumes of Chōei's collected works in 1930–31.

The first article to appear in English on Chōei was published in 1913. Written just one year after the Meiji Emperor's death, it depicted Chōei as a harbinger of the Meiji sovereign's "reign of enlightenment."[67] Despite some inaccuracies, this early paper is still worth reading, particularly for the translation of Chōei's 1838 *The Tale of a Dream.* The fact that such a detailed piece was written at so early a date is testimony to the intrinsic interest that Chōei's story held for people living at the end of the Meiji era.

Much of the Japanese scholarship written after this came under the influence of the larger debate about the historical significance of *rangaku* outlined above. There is evidence of the influence of these arguments in English scholarship too, for they were of great interest to modernization theorists as well as to Marxist historians. In 1950, the eminent English scholar of Japan, G. B. Sansom, included a section on Kazan and Chōei in his *The Western World and Japan.* As one might expect from its title, "Forerunners of the Restoration Movement," Sansom too saw the pair as enlightened, though tragically oppressed, figures on the eve of the Meiji restoration.[68]

---

66. Takano Chōun, *Takano Chōei den*, pp. 3–4.
67. Greene, "Life of Takano Nagahide," p. 456.
68. Sansom, *The Western World and Japan*, pp. 262–89.

This view began to be challenged with the publication in 1951 of W. G. Beasley's *Great Britain and the Opening of Japan*. Like Sansom, Beasley included a very brief account of Chōei and Kazan; but he was careful to point out that despite their criticism of the "shell and repel" edict, both men still believed that trade with Western countries should be refused.[69] This clarification came with a reminder that *rangaku* scholars, like other intellectual groups, continued to see foreigners as "predatory and degenerate." The reminder was reiterated in 1986 by Goodman[70] and also by Wakabayashi, who characterized Chōei as a xenophobe.[71]

Scholarship on the life of Chōei cannot be considered complete without the work of Satō Shōsuke (introduced above). Satō's work is particularly interesting for the way it presented challenges to popularly held ideas about Chōei. His work was designed to correct what he saw as the biases of earlier works, and he believed he could do this by an objective analysis of primary documents.

One of the most important challenges Satō made was to question Chōei's image as a political figure and his role in the events of the 1839 repression. Chōei and Kazan (who was his employer and mentor) had typically been seen more or less equally as targets in the events of the repression and as having similar ways of thinking about foreign affairs. In response to this, Satō argued that they were quite different. Kazan was a statesman and administrator with a sophisticated vision of foreign affairs, while Chōei was primarily a physician and scientist, who under Kazan's influence after 1832 had become interested in broader political and social issues.[72]

Kazan himself wrote figuratively of Chōei's political awareness that he was "no more than a corporal" and was "not yet ready to become a general."[73] This is hardly surprising when one considers that Chōei's training was in medicine, while Kazan was a trained politician with responsibility for coastal defense in his domain.

---

69. Beasley, *Great Britain and the Opening of Japan, 1834–1858*, p. 35.
70. Goodman, *Japan: The Dutch Experience*, p. 210.
71. Wakabayashi, *Anti-Foreignism*, p. 61.
72. Satō, ed., *Watanabe Kazan, Takano Chōei*, pp. 59–60.
73. Quoted in ibid., p. 86.

In a detailed study of the events surrounding the repression,[74] Satō argued that they were largely the result of a personal and professional grudge held against Kazan by a particular Bakufu official. Every story needs a villain, and this man, by the name of Torii Yōzō (1815–74), is often demonized as the great enemy of Western learning and progress in late Tokugawa Japan. This was partly because he was the son of Hayashi Jussai, head of the Bakufu's Confucian school, and this fitted the idea of the *bansha no goku* being a clash between the old establishment and the new form of learning. In fact, Torii was probably just carrying out orders in his role as a *metsuke* (inspector). His instructions were to find out the author of *The Tale of a Dream,* and although his investigations were rather bungled, this is basically what he achieved. In the course of the investigation, drafts of Kazan's *Shinkiron* (A case for restraint) and other manuscripts critical of Bakufu policy were found at Kazan's home, and it was on the basis of these that he and Chōei, who gave himself up, were prosecuted. Although it is probably fair to say that Torii was no friend of Western learning, the events of 1839 perhaps had more to do with the government's concern about public criticism than with Torii's personal ambitions.[75]

Satō, therefore, is probably incorrect to argue that Kazan was the only intended victim of the repression. As the author of a critical piece of literature, Chōei was placing himself in a dangerous position, no matter what his connection to Western learning. Nevertheless, it does seem fair to say that *The Tale of a Dream* was not at all representative of his work as a whole. Most of Chōei's work was in medicine, science, and social welfare. Moreover, as Satō points out, *The Tale of a Dream* was not even a very sophisticated piece of work compared to Kazan's *A Case for Restraint.*[76] It is interesting to consider, in the light of these reflections, the following passage from Chōei's *Wasuregatami* (A memento), which

---

74. Satō's writings on the *bansha no goku* are numerous. Perhaps the most accessible account is the 1997 *Takano Chōei.*

75. I am indebted to Mitani, "Rekishi no hotei," for this interpretation.

76. A translation of Chōei's *Yume monogatari* can be found in Greene's "Life of Takano Nagahide," pp. 423–30. Kazan's *Shinkiron* has been translated by Bonnie Abiko in the appendix of her thesis: "Watanabe Kazan: The Man and His Times," pp. 293–304.

was written in prison to proclaim his innocence. A possible reading seems to be that the "*rangaku*" to which Chōei refers means his usual translation work on medicine, and that he did not consider *The Tale of a Dream* to be *rangaku* at all: "If one were to take *rangaku* as one's life's work and die for it, one would be loyal in both deeds and death. Thus, there would be nothing to resent in terms of reason, and in terms of virtue nothing of which to be ashamed. However, I could not but regret dying for the sake of my *Tale of a Dream*."[77] Thus, while the events of the "imprisonment of barbarian associates" in 1839 had a profound effect, both on *rangaku* in general and on the course of Chōei's life as an individual, it would appear that writing political commentary was by no means what he considered his work to be.

The study of the life of Chōei has been popular because he was seen as a martyr to the process of modernization. The tragedy of his unfulfilled life and of his fate as a victim of politics cannot be denied. To focus purely on the tragedy, however, is to forget the triumph of his role as one of the most talented *rangaku* scholars of his time. It is therefore one of the concerns of this book to return to the period before Chōei's arrest in order to examine his place in history, not as a political victim, nor as part of a narrative of modernization, but as a *rangaku* scholar and doctor.

Chōei and Takahashi Keisaku

During the 1830s, Chōei built up a warm relationship with three doctors, Fukuda Sōtei (1791–1840), Yanagida Teizō (1795–1855), and Takahashi Keisaku (1799–1875), in the province of Kōzuke. The villages around the post town of Nakanojō, with their mountain herbs and thermal springs, formed an interesting geographical setting for this network of physicians. In return for their financial patronage, Chōei shared with them his knowledge of *rangaku* scholarship. They eventually wrote together two collaborative works on famine and disease, utilizing Western knowledge in order to approach a local problem. This is a perfect example of how Japa-

---

77. Takano Chōei, "Wasuregatami," p. 182.

nese doctors, even in rural areas, actively sought Western knowledge to serve their practical needs.

The two documents, *Kyūkō nibutsukō* (Treatise on two things for the relief of famine) and *Hieki yōhō* (Methods of avoiding epidemic diseases), were written in 1836, at the height of the Tenpō famine. They formed part of a wider debate about famine in Tokugawa Japan and demonstrate the influential idea that Western learning was of practical benefit. As will be seen, in some instances the documents contain quite surprising misinterpretations. These kinds of errors have often been judged in intellectual histories as a "failure" to understand Western knowledge correctly. However, they by no means detract from the meaning of their arguments in their own time and place.

Chōei did not merely translate what he read in Dutch books, but tried to interpret and apply this knowledge to problems facing his own society: in this case, the issues of starvation and epidemic disease around the time of the Tenpō famine. The question is not the extent to which he understood on its own terms the Western knowledge he read, but what he did with that knowledge on his terms. Even when dealing with medical concepts, it was necessary for Chōei to put them into a form in which they could be readily accepted and understood. This task was made easier by a basic compatibility between some of the concepts in Japanese versions of Chinese medicine, particularly *koihō*, and Western medicine of the time. By considering these documents in their social context, it is possible to see the study of *rangaku* not as a failure, but as a creative and practical adaptation. It becomes easier to understand *why* knowledge was interpreted in certain ways. Finally, it becomes possible to place Chōei in an unusual light: not a political activist, but a socially conscious doctor of medicine.

An analysis of the diary of Takahashi Keisaku provides a further example of the way in which Western knowledge was reaching rural Japan. It helps to establish the role of members of the rural elite in facilitating the spread of medical and other knowledge through their social networks. At the same time, it creates a valuable portrait of the everyday life of a country doctor of the Edo period, a subject about which very little is known.

Keisaku's diary is a rich source of information, not only about his daily life but also about his personal networks. Keisaku was a village official and a keen poet, in addition to his work as a medical doctor. Despite his rural environment in Kōzuke, he was far from isolated. In addition to the acquaintances he made in the course of his official duties, his connections with other doctors, poets, and local intellectuals kept him supplied with a constant stream of visitors, from both near and far.

Historians have already pointed to the importance of social networks in Japanese contexts. For example, it has been shown that villagers living on the outskirts of Edo used large regional networks for administrative and political purposes. These networks were formed by village elites, whose roles as wealthy farmers, businessmen, and community leaders were notably "often played by one and the same person."[78] The social and familial networks of the rural elite, which ranged over a wide geographical area, helped to create a kind of class solidarity that formed the basis for the business, religious, political, and leisured activities of the rural entrepreneurs.[79]

Social networks also appear to have been significant in terms of the technological history of Japan. According to Morris-Suzuki, a network of productive centers arose during the Edo period that created a "dynamism and flexibility" that helped to determine the way Japanese society coped with the sudden influx of Western technology at the end of the nineteenth century.[80]

This network of productive centers was especially important in the countryside. There, producers were free from the limitations of urban guilds, a factor that "encouraged the diffusion of technology and skills."[81] Importantly, in association with this trend, there arose a class of wealthy farmers, "often with a substantial interest

78. Anne Walthall, "Village Networks Sōdai and the Sale of Edo Nightsoil," p. 303.

79. Anne Walthall, "The Family Ideology of the Rural Entrepreneurs in Nineteenth Century Japan," p. 469.

80. Morris-Suzuki, *The Technological Transformation*, p. 34.

81. Ibid., p. 21.

in craft industry, who had both the time and the capital to try out new techniques."[82]

It is significant that authors should trace the importance of social networks for a particular class of rural elite. The rural entrepreneurs, or *gōnō*, with their curious status between ordinary peasants and the samurai ruling class, have been the object of much historical attention. Not only have they been credited with an important role in the diffusion and development of technology, they have also been recognized in a more general economic sense as carriers of Japan's modern economic transformation.[83] If medicine may be thought of as "technology," it may be supposed that the networks of the *gōnō* had a similar role to play in the spread of medical techniques. Just as rural elites experimented with new technologies in areas such as silk production, they may have had the time, education, and courage to try new forms of medicine. By scouring Keisaku's diary for evidence of the number and nature of his personal networks, it is possible to draw a picture not only of his sophisticated social life but of the way technological and medical information came to reach rural Kōzuke.

Western Knowledge and Medical Lives

Takano Chōei was a self-made man. In the beginning, he was nothing more than the son of a middle-ranking samurai doctor in the village of Mizusawa in the province of Mutsu in northern Japan. His move to Edo and the constant struggle he faced there to make a living as a town doctor and medical scholar tell us a great deal about the study and practice of medicine in early modern Japan. Social aspects such as these have been much neglected in the history of Japanese medicine.

The following chapter begins with a short biography of Chōei based on the sources discussed in the historiographical section above, followed by an examination of medical education in the Tokugawa period. This second section uses the letters Chōei wrote as a young man, together with a number of Japanese secondary

---

82. Ibid.
83. Pratt, *Japan's Protoindustrial Elite.*

sources. Finally, the different kinds of doctors and their social statuses are addressed. This last section relies heavily on evidence found in humorous poems of the Edo period, which have been collected in a recent book.[84] These short, gently humorous verses were part of the culture of urban commoners, though increasingly they were enjoyed by members of the warrior class too.[85] They often contained direct observations of everyday life and are therefore an especially valuable source of information about the everyday history of medicine, which so often remained unrecorded elsewhere.

The Kōzuke physicians, their environment, and the way in which they shared knowledge with Chōei is the subject of Chapter 2, drawing on a combination of local historical materials and secondary sources in English. In addition to the study of this community of rural physicians and their environment, the chapter attempts to link their lives to broader changes in contemporary society. I draw upon a range of scholarship, both in English and in Japanese, which provides clues to the nature of life in Japan in the first half of the nineteenth century. The past decade or so has seen a number of studies in English on life in Tokugawa Japan.[86] This section brings this wealth of recent scholarship in English together with the local history so carefully undertaken by Japanese historians. This serves two purposes: to assist in hypothesizing about the social and geographical conditions that allowed the Kōzuke physicians to live the lives they did and to add a dimension of social history to documentary local histories of *rangaku*.

Chapter 3 is a detailed study of the collaborative works *Treatise on Two Things for the Relief of Famine* and *Methods of Avoiding Epi-*

---

84. Ono, *Edo no machiisha*.

85. Kato, *A History of Japanese Literature*, p. 209.

86. These works include both short and long general overviews by Nakane, Jansen, and Totman, a meticulous study of travel by Vaporis, and works on standards of living and material culture by Hanley. Relating to medicine, there is Johnston's study of tuberculosis and Jannetta's work on epidemics. See Nakane and Oishi, eds., *Tokugawa Japan*; Jansen, "Japan in the Early Nineteenth Century"; Totman, *Early Modern Japan*; Vaporis, *Breaking Barriers*; Hanley, "Tokugawa Society: Material Culture, Standard of Living, and Life-styles"; idem, *Everyday Things In Premodern Japan*; Jannetta, *Epidemics and Mortality in Early Modern Japan*; and Johnston, *The Modern Epidemic*.

demic Diseases. Full English translations of each document appear in the Appendix. The chapter also contains excerpts from Yanagida Teizō's diary, which vividly describe the local effects of the famine in Kōzuke.

Chapter 4 is a study of the life and work of Takahashi Keisaku, based on his diary. It provides both a picture of the life of a rural doctor and a means of thinking about the role of elite villagers in the spread of information. As Keisaku lived on into the Meiji period, it also allows us to reflect on the change from the study of *rangaku* to the modern scientific study of medicine thereafter, and how doctors coped when faced with the intellectual gap between the two.

All of the chapters are connected in some way to Takano Chōei. They are also interwoven with some recurring themes: the practical nature of Western learning and its influence as a catalyst for social change; the spread of information and literacy; rural elites; the social role of doctors and their daily lives. This book suggests that Western knowledge was not some kind of immutable entity that had to be absorbed as a whole in order to be of use. Instead, it was received in a piecemeal fashion and creatively adapted to fit the existing intellectual framework. Scholars such as Chōei went to enormous lengths to obtain such knowledge, not only for the sake of their own intellectual curiosity but also for what they saw as its practical benefits for the society in which they lived. Nor was scientific exchange restricted to elite scholars who were based in the political and economic centers. Those on the geographic margins of society were active participants too. If the acceptance of new knowledge by a society is measured by its ultimate domestication and permeation into everyday life, then ordinary provincial scholars cannot be left out of the picture. While literacy and the publication of books were vitally important to the dispersal of new information, the significance of social networks in the spread of such knowledge should not be overlooked. Local medical practitioners, with pivotal roles in village social networks, contributed vitally to this intellectual activity.

CHAPTER I

Takano Chōei and the
Medical Arena

The extraordinary life of Takano Chōei (1804–50) reads more like a historical novel than the biography of a medical practitioner. A brilliant scholar who, at the height of his career, was made a political prisoner, Chōei staged a dramatic escape and lived for several years as a fugitive before finally committing suicide when he was at last recaptured. What can the study of such an unusual man reveal about the workings of medicine in nineteenth-century Japanese society?

As one of the leading scholars of Western learning in the first half of the nineteenth century, Chōei is worthy of attention for this reason alone. His academic training made him part of an elite group whose members studied with the finest teachers of Western medicine, including Philipp Franz von Siebold (1796–1866) in Nagasaki. Socially, however, Chōei was always a marginal figure. As a student, he perpetually struggled to pay his fees, and as an adult he relied on the patronage of his friends to help him make a living and introduce him to influential scholarly circles. As a non-elite medical practitioner, the social relationships that Chōei maintained are of particular interest in providing clues to the reception and practice of Western medicine in early modern Japan.

Moreover, Chōei left detailed records of his life as a young medical student in Edo, which are extremely helpful in creating a picture of how students lived and trained. After beginning with a short biography, this chapter will use those letters to examine his life within the context of the broader medical scene. The picture of the training and social status of doctors, the different types of medical practitioners, and the relationships between various groups in the nineteenth-century medical arena is filled in by using humorous poems about doctors current in Chōei's day.

Takano Chōei

Takano Chōei, who was known as Kyōsai during his early life, was born in 1804 in Mizusawa in the province of Mutsu (present-day Iwate prefecture).[1] He was the third son of Gotō Sōsuke, a middle-ranking samurai. As a young boy, however, he was adopted by his uncle Takano Gensai, with the intention that he would eventually marry his cousin Chio and become head of the Takano family. This was a common practice that helped families without sons to continue their family lines. Gensai was a doctor, and Chōei quickly came under a conspicuous medical influence. His uncle had studied under Sugita Genpaku (1733–1817), that pioneer famous for opening up the study of Western medicine in Japan. Chōei's grandfather had also traveled to Kyoto as a youth to study medicine. Growing up with these well-trained physicians as examples, it is hardly surprising that Chōei should have followed in their footsteps. Indeed, it was probably expected of him, as medical practices were in many cases hereditary. His medical schooling seems to have begun at an early age; he received basic training from his grandfather and from a local doctor of Chinese medicine.

In 1820, Chōei traveled with his elder brother Tansai and cousin Yōrin to Edo to study medicine. According to family legend, it was only with great reluctance that Gensai let him go, for he was not in a position to spend much money on his adopted son's education. Although Gensai served his domain as an official doctor and received a stipend, it was a mere five and a half *koku*, and he

---

1. Unless otherwise stated, this biography is based on details recorded in Takano Chōun, *Takano Chōei den*.

was by no means a rich man.[2] It was only after Chōei won some money in a lottery that he was finally able to have his way.[3] Gensai was right to be fearful of sending his adopted son away, for as we shall see, Chōei never came back to fulfill his filial obligations.

Upon arriving in Edo, Chōei had some difficulty finding a teacher, but he finally managed to persuade a reluctant Sugita Hakugen, heir to the famous Genpaku, to take him as a day student. This arrangement lasted only a year, for Chōei soon left to study with Yoshida Chōshuku (1779–1824). It seems he enjoyed a much better relationship with his new teacher, for it was Chōshuku who gave him the name "Chōei" in 1822. It included a character from Chōshuku's own name, as a measure of the regard in which he was held.[4] Chōshuku had trained with Katsuragawa Hoshū (1751–1809), one of the early leading scholars of Western medicine. Chōshuku was also one of the first doctors to prescribe Western methods for internal medicine at a time when Western medical practice in Japan was largely restricted to surgery. Sadly, however, Chōshuku suddenly became ill and died in 1824.[5] The sudden death of his teacher shocked Chōei "beyond words," and it seems to have spurred him to continue his education in Nagasaki the next year.

Chōei's journey to Nagasaki took place in 1825, after a short spell working as a replacement teacher in Chōshuku's school. Since his teacher had died without appointing a successor, Chōei and his fellow students were anxious to make sure that his school did not fall into ruin.[6] Chōei told his adoptive father of his decision to go to Nagasaki only after he had already departed. He did so in a letter requesting that Gensai repay the loan he had taken out in order to cover his travel expenses. The long-suffering Gensai no doubt repaid the loan, but Chōei's impudence appears to have upset him

---

2. Satō, *Takano Chōei*, p. 9. A *koku* was about five bales of rice and was considered to be enough rice to feed an adult for a year.

3. See Takano Chōun, *Takano Chōei den*, pp. 58–60. It appears that Chōei's elder brother Gotō Tansai was to be adopted by Sakano Chōan, the local doctor of Chinese medicine, and was presumably funded by him.

4. Takano Chōun, *Takano Chōei den*, p. 88.

5. Takano Chōei Kinenkan, ed., *Takano Chōei no tegami*, p. 73.

6. Ibid., pp. 76–77.

so much that he never wrote to his adopted son again. Evidence for this can be seen in a New Year's letter Chōei wrote in 1827, the year in which Gensai died:

Since the year before last I have had no way of knowing your circumstances and can do nothing but spend my time worrying night and day. With the days and months a blur, already three springs have passed. I surmise it is entirely because you disapprove of my studying in Nagasaki. Now, after all this time, there is nothing that can be done, and I pray a hundred prayers that you will forgive me.[7]

When the news of his adoptive father's death reached him, Chōei was on a visit to the islands of Iki and Tsushima, collecting medicinal herbs.[8] Claiming that he was ill, he did not return home to take up the position of head of the family, as duty required.

Chōei's purpose in going to Nagasaki in 1825 was to study at Siebold's school, the Narutakijuku. Siebold was an acclaimed German physician and scholar, who first arrived in Japan to work at the Dutch compound in 1823. His task, given him by the governor-general of the Dutch East Indies, was to learn as much about Japan as possible and, in exchange, to teach European medicine to the Japanese.[9]

Students gathered at the Narutakijuku from all over the country, because this was the first time that Japanese students were able to receive systematic training in Western medicine from a European. The school, which was located on shore in the Narutaki area of Nagasaki, was open from 1824 to 1828, during which time Siebold was permitted by the Nagasaki town magistrate to go there once a week to teach and to perform various other medical duties in the town. In conjunction with his lectures in Dutch, he also taught by demonstration, which was something of a revelation in contemporary teaching practices.[10] There is evidence in the records kept by a student who was studying at another school in Nagasaki that Siebold came to the school to carry out at least six surgical opera-

---

7. Ibid., pp. 105–6.
8. Satō, *Takano Chōei*, p. 46.
9. Beukers, *The Mission of Hippocrates*, p. 22.
10. Ibid., p. 58.

tions.[11] They included cases of a buildup of fluid in the scrotum, hemorrhoids, cancer and inflammation of the throat, and a lipoma (a type of benign tumor) in a twelve-year-old boy. According to this account, Chōei was among the students from Siebold's school who came to view this operation.

Siebold's activities have traditionally been given great prominence in accounts of the introduction of Western medicine to Japan. The case of this young boy, however, is a poignant example of the extent to which Siebold's medical activities were effectively restricted by official regulations. After the operation, Siebold was obliged to entrust the care of the patient to his Japanese students, and return to his home on the island of Dejima. Some time afterwards, the boy took a turn for the worse and developed a headache and fever, eventually losing consciousness. The students rushed to ask their teacher's advice, but they were not allowed to visit Dejima at night, so even in this emergency they were forced to send messages back and forth about how to proceed. Despite their best efforts, the young boy died.[12] Much of the teaching at Siebold's school, too, seems to have been done by his senior students.[13] From the start, the students were obliged to take much of the responsibility for their own learning.

Some of the students who studied under Siebold were allowed to board at the school, the requisite conditions being that they were both talented and very poor. It has been suggested that this was because such students were not in a position to refuse to undertake projects for their teacher, even should the work involve something dangerous or unlawful.[14] Chōei was one such student. Siebold's pupils were expected to write reports about Japan in lieu of school fees. Chōei's essays are the most numerous of all those remaining; his work covered such diverse subjects as flower arrang-

---

11. The student's name was Miyahara Ryōseki, and he was studying at the school of Yoshio Kōsai.

12. Aoki, *Zaison rangaku no kenkyū*, pp. 243–50. A brief account of this operation also appears in Beukers, *The Mission of Hippocrates*, p. 78.

13. Satō, *Takano Chōei*, pp. 30–31.

14. Satō, *Yōgakushi ronkō*, p. 151.

ing, the manners of Japanese women, temples in Kyoto, and the cultivation of tea.[15]

During this period, Chōei, whose Dutch-language skills were already highly regarded, supplemented his income by writing translations. It has been suggested that he began working on the major medical works he published in the early 1830s, such as his *Fundamentals of Western Medicine*, while still in Nagasaki.[16]

His peaceful days of study came to an abrupt end, however, in 1828, because of a turn of events that has come to be known as the "Siebold Affair."[17] After several successful years of research, which had included a visit to Edo with the official Dutch procession in 1826,[18] Siebold had been preparing to leave with his collection of Japanese paraphernalia. He had, however, in the course of his research, aroused the suspicions of the Bakufu authorities. The main source of concern was his relationship with the respected Japanese astronomer Takahashi Kageyasu (1785–1829). When Siebold visited Edo, he met Kageyasu, who gave him a copy of a recent and very accurate map of Japan in return for some Western books and maps.[19] When Bakufu officials discovered that the two had been secretly corresponding, eventually the matter of the map also came to light. It was strictly forbidden to engage in direct correspondence with a foreigner, let alone to hand over something as important to the national interest as a map. Kageyasu was arrested late in 1828. The Siebold Affair has often been ascribed to a typhoon that struck Nagasaki in the tenth month of 1828 and forced Siebold to unload the contents of the ship and have them inspected. According to this view, the secret map was then discovered and traced to Kageyasu. Recent research, however, has shown that in fact there

---

15. See Takano Chōei Zenshū Kankō Kai, ed., *Takano Chōei zenshū*, vol. 6.

16. Satō, *Takano Chōei*, p. 42.

17. See Keene, *The Japanese Discovery*, pp. 147–55.

18. Siebold's account of the journey is available in Japanese in Kure Shūzō, ed., *Shiiboruto Edo sanpu kikō*. It is also summarized in Bowers, *Western Medical Pioneers*, pp. 116–23.

19. The map was a copy of that made by Inō Tadataka (1745–1818), who is celebrated for producing the first accurate map of Japan, from Ezo in the north to Kyushu in the south.

was nothing on board the boat when the typhoon hit. The source of the investigation can instead be traced to Kageyasu in Edo.[20] Kageyasu was sent to prison, where he fell ill and died. Siebold was confined, investigated, and eventually expelled in 1829. Some of Siebold's students were punished by being exiled from Nagasaki or prevented from entering the capital, Edo. The Narutaki school was completely shut down.

Siebold fulfilled a dream by managing to return to Japan in 1859, but it was a fruitless time and he was ousted in 1861 by European diplomats, who found him disruptive. He returned to Germany again but is said to have never stopped yearning for Japan. He made an enormous contribution to European knowledge of Japan, through the books he published and his impressive collections of Japanese material culture.[21] Incidentally, his daughter Ine (1827–1903) by his Japanese mistress remained in Japan and went on to study medicine herself.[22]

Upon hearing of his teacher's detention, Chōei, probably fearing that he too would be incriminated, fled to Kumamoto. He then made his way slowly, via Hirose Tansō's (1782–1856) famous school, the Kangien in Hida, to Kyoto. In Kyoto, he treated patients, gave some lectures, and made efforts to meet several prominent Kyoto physicians of Western medicine.[23] Finally, in a letter to his family in 1830, Chōei declared that he was ill and was unable to return home. It was a transparent excuse, however, for in the same letter he described his new research plans and wrote that, in order to carry out the work he intended to do, he needed to be in Edo: "Edo being the place where I studied for several years, I have many close friends there, and it is a good place to recover from my sick-

---

20. Ōba, *Hana no otoko Shiiboruto*, pp. 84–89.

21. For more detail on the career of Siebold in English, see Bowers, *Western Medical Pioneers*, pp. 92–173; Beukers, *The Mission of Hippocrates*; and Fukui et al., *Siebold's Japan*.

22. Sōda, *Zusetsu Nihon iryō bunkashi*, p. 248. See also Beukers, *The Mission of Hippocrates*, pp. 124–32.

23. Such as Fujibayashi Taisuke (1781–1836), Komori Tou (1782–1843), Koishi Genzui (1784–1849), and Shingū Ryōtei (1787–1854).

ness. It is also a good place to be employed in the service of my homeland."[24]

Chōei returned to Edo toward the end of 1830 and opened a school, the Daikandō, in the Kōjimachi area. In refusing to return home to his family in Mizusawa, he spurned his cousin Chio and cut himself off from his samurai status and stipend. Thus he became a *machiisha*, a common town doctor.

Of his decision to settle in Edo, Chōei explained:

Consequently, it is difficult for me now, because of my poor health, to learn techniques, and for myself, I would like to devote the rest of my life exclusively to study. By doing this, I will be considered to be of no use to my lord, and all these years of study to have been to no purpose: a shameful situation. If possible I hope to serve by some other means, at least to repay one ten-millionth of the favor from which I have benefited. When I thought so hard that I forgot to eat and sleep, I selected one aspect of Western learning. Unless I am in Edo, it will be difficult for me to undertake this work. This is no ordinary undertaking, and . . . when it is completed, it will probably benefit all of Mizusawa and of course too I hope, those in authority.[25]

The "one aspect of Western learning" to which Chōei refers is probably a reference to physiology, the subject of his major work, *Seisetsu igen sūyō* (Fundamentals of Western medicine). This was the first comprehensive work in Japanese on Western physiology.[26] The first volume was in five parts, of which only the first was published in 1832. The other parts were circulated in manuscript form. Little is known about the second volume, which is no longer extant.

The first part of volume 1 contained sections on the distinguishing features of living beings, and on the differences between humans and animals and between the human races. This was followed by an overview of the human body (solids, liquids, vital power, spiritual power, and inherited character). Part two discussed the various functions of different parts of the body, the senses, sleep,

---

24. Takano Chōei Kinenkan, ed., *Takano Chōei no tegami*, p. 124.

25. Ibid., p. 123.

26. Fujikawa, *Nihon igakushi kōyō*, 2: 99. The first volume is reprinted in full in Takano Chōei Zenshū Kankō Kai, ed., *Takano Chōei zenshū*, 1: 5–106.

and the physiology of movement. Part three concerned circulation, breathing, and secretions. Part four dealt with digestion, absorption, blood production, body temperature, and excretion. The fifth part covered the reproductive organs, fertilization, nutrition of the fetus, and the physiology of childbirth. The work was based on Dutch translations of works in German by Blumenbach (1752–1840) and T. G. A. Roose (1771–1803) and in French by Georges de la Faye (1699–1781).[27] It was the publication of part one of this book that made Chōei's name as a scholar.

The next few years were to be the most stable and productive of Chōei's life. It was during this period that he came under the influence of Watanabe Kazan (1793–1841), the man who was in many ways to share his fate.[28] Kazan was born in Edo as the son of a highly ranked but poor samurai of the Tahara domain (present-day Aichi). He lived most of his life in the daimyo's official residence in the capital, where he was trained as a Confucian statesman and as an artist. Due to the domain's failing economy, Kazan was forced as a youth to sell his artwork to help support his family. Gradually, as he rose to a high rank in the Tahara bureaucracy, he became interested in famine, agricultural reform, and the military defense of the domain's coastline. It was in his role as an administrator, therefore, that he turned to Western learning for inspiration.

It is probable that Kazan and Chōei met in 1832. The area in which Chōei lived in Kōjimachi was very close to the Tahara domain residence, and Kazan, who could not read Dutch, asked Chōei to translate for him, arranging for the indigent scholar to be paid a small salary by the domain. Koseki San'ei, who had also studied under Yoshida Chōshuku, and another scholar by the name of Hatasaki Kanae, were similarly employed.[29] Soon, Chōei began to participate in a study group that Kazan also attended. This was called the Shōshikai and was a gathering of intellectuals

---

27. Miyashita, "A Bibliography of the Dutch Medical Books Translated into Japanese," pp. 18–19.

28. A detailed study of Kazan's life and career may be found in Bonnie Abiko, "Watanabe Kazan: The Man and His Times."

29. Satō, ed., *Watanabe Kazan, Takano Chōei*, p. 53.

and officials interested in Western learning and foreign affairs.[30] The immediate reason for creating the group seems to have been to discuss problems of famine, which afflicted the country throughout the 1830s. Although details are sketchy, there is evidence that the group evolved into a medium for the exchange of new information, with a particular emphasis on Western learning.[31]

It was also during the early 1830s that Chōei began to associate closely with three physicians from the province of Kōzuke (present-day Gunma). As will be outlined in the following chapter, their association was to be characterized by a number of visits, warm exchanges by letter, both social and academic in nature, and financial support from the doctors for Chōei's publications. In addition, it led to the collaborative works *Kyūkō nibutsukō* (Treatise on two things for the relief of famine) and *Hieki yōhō* (Methods of avoiding epidemic diseases), both published in 1837.

Another important person to figure in the writing of these works was Uchida Yatarō (1805–82), who signed himself as the "scribe" of both documents. Unlike Chōei's students in Kōzuke, Yatarō chose to use his Dutch-language skills as a means to study mathematics rather than medicine. By the time the Meiji government decided to implement the Western calendar in 1872, he was head of the Meiji calendrical office.[32] Yatarō was probably one of Chōei's most trusted students. It was he who looked after Chōei's wife and family during the years he spent in prison and who was

---

30. The group had been founded by Endō Katsusuke (1789–1851), a Confucian scholar who had become friendly with Kazan through his literary interests. Literally, Shōshikai means "Age Veneration Society," and as a generic term, it means a society of elderly people interested in poetry and the arts. It is not certain why this name was chosen for the group.

31. Satō, *Yōgakushi kenkyū josetsu*, pp. 134–35. There has been some confusion about the membership of the Shōshikai and the extent to which it was a politically motivated group. I have followed Satō, who saw it purely as a study group and argued that Chōei's later assertions about its political nature were exaggerated. An alternative interpretation may be found in H. D. Harootunian, "Late Tokugawa Culture and Thought," pp. 231–52.

32. Sugimoto and Swain, *Science and Culture in Traditional Japan*, pp. 345–46, 360.

probably responsible for creating an opportunity for Chōei to work secretly for the Uwajima domain after his escape.[33]

Chōei married a woman by the name of Yuki in 1838. Little is known about her background, which has meant that scholars have speculated freely about her, some suggesting, for example, that she was a geisha.[34] Chōei was not long married, however, before his life was turned upside down by his writing that year of *Bojutsu yume monogatari* (The tale of a dream).[35] This piece was written in 1838 to protest against the "shell and repel" edict. The events of the *bansha no goku* (imprisonment of barbarian associates) began with the arrest in 1839 of Watanabe Kazan, who was suspected of writing *The Tale of a Dream* and of plotting to set up a colony on the Ogasawara Islands. Chōei turned himself in to the city magistrate shortly afterward.[36] Upon hearing of Kazan's arrest, Koseki San'ei, who had also translated work for Kazan, feared his own implication and committed suicide.[37] Kazan also eventually took his own life, while under house arrest in Tahara.

Chōei's status as an ex-samurai meant that he was dealt a harsher punishment than his employer, Kazan. Far from a relatively comfortable house arrest, Chōei spent five years in the commoners' section of the Kodenmachō prison in Edo, where

neither sunlight penetrated, nor the wind circulated and where several people were squeezed in close together like fish-scales. The smell of sickness and squalor combined to form a strange stench, and because every corner of the prison was filled with it, the odor was indescribable. . . . Furthermore, people who up until the day before had been healthy would fall down ill the following morning and die.[38]

---

33. Satō, *Takano Chōei*, p. 164.

34. See Nakamura, "A Portrait of Takano Chōei."

35. *Bojutsu* refers to the year in which it was written. A translation of Chōei's *Yume monogatari* is found in Greene, "Life of Takano Nagahide," pp. 390–492. Kazan's *Shinkiron* has been translated in Abiko, "Watanabe Kazan: The Man and His Times," pp. 293–304.

36. See Satō, *Watanabe Kazan, Takano Chōei*, pp. 60–80.

37. Satō, *Takano Chōei*, pp. 105–6.

38. Takano Chōei, "Wasuregatami," p. 177.

Chōei's circumstances in the prison were, however, better than those of many of the other inmates. A sentence of life imprisonment was actually quite unusual; most inmates could expect to be either released or executed. It is thought that Chōei escaped execution only because he had turned himself in to the authorities. As a long-term prisoner and as a medical doctor with valuable skills, he was therefore in a unique position. It was not long before he became the *rōnanushi* (prison leader), which was the highest office among the inmates. He received a raised platform of ten *tatami* mats from which he could keep an eye on all the others. His job was to help the prison officials maintain order, to see that rules were obeyed, and to prevent prisoners from running away or committing suicide. He also had certain privileges, such as being able to obtain forbidden items, gamble, smoke, and so on.[39] Furthermore, Chōei's status appears to have assisted him in maintaining contact with the outside world. After becoming *rōnanushi*, he was able to send letters and money to his friends and family.[40] When new prisoners entered the prison, it was customary for them to bring with them about ten *ryō* (quite a large sum of money). This would be divided among the inmate officers, and the *rōnanushi* would, of course, receive the most.[41] Thus, ironically, Chōei had more money than he had ever enjoyed before while in prison. His high status in the prison also no doubt assisted him in his plans for escape.

The letters Chōei wrote while in prison suggest that, with the help of various supporters, he was at first engaged in attempts to arrange a pardon. The custom was for such appeals to be made by the relatives of prisoners at Kan'eiji temple in Ueno, because when memorial services were held there for members of the shogunal family, some amnesties were usually granted. The priests would make up a list of prisoners and forward it to the Bakufu, where

---

39. Kokushi Daijiten Henshū Iinkai, ed., *Kokushi daijiten,* 14: 777.

40. See Takano Chōei Kinenkan, ed., *Takano Chōei no tegami,* p. 159. Most of the letters were addressed to his cousin Mogi Kyōichirō. Others were addressed to a man called Yonekichi, who had been in prison with Chōei and was released. He appears to have helped Chōei in his communications with the outside world.

41. Satō, *Yōgakushi ronkō,* p. 173.

upon bureaucrats would decide who should be pardoned. Since Chōei's crime was a political one, he had next to no chance of being freed in this manner.[42] Nevertheless, in a letter of 1842, he wrote about arranging for a friend to put his name on the amnesty list. The following year, he appears instead to have decided to earn favor in other ways. He wrote of making an application to undertake official translations and treat the sick in the government's labor camp. Suddenly, however, in 1844, he became much more secretive, and although he had always displayed an optimistic attitude in his letters regarding his release from prison, the following passage, from a letter written to a friend and ex-inmate, does indeed seem to be a covert reference to his plans for escape:

This year there are many things that I am going to request. Even if just one of them is granted, I will have something on which to rely for the future. I think that probably at least one of them will be granted, and this being so, eventually I will be able to see you again. . . . I am still well and do not intend to die with things as they are. . . . In summer I hope to be given my freedom.[43]

Chōei made his escape in the early hours of the morning on the thirtieth of the sixth month, 1844.[44] It was a moonless night in summer. Taking advantage of a rule that in the event of a fire, prisoners were released for three days, Chōei arranged for a menial worker by the name of Eizō to set fire to the prison. As anticipated, the prisoners were released on the condition that they gather again at the Ekōin temple or the city magistrate's office, depending on the direction of the wind.[45] Those who returned would have their sentences reduced. Chōei, of course, did not return. Two days before this, his close friend Suzuki Shunzan, who had been working in his native Tahara, suddenly returned to Edo. Shunzan would later help Chōei find somewhere to live and have him help with the translation of a military book.[46]

---

42. Ibid., p. 174.
43. Takano Chōei Kinenkan, ed., *Takano Chōei no tegami*, pp. 217–19.
44. Satō, *Yōgakushi ronkō*, p. 181.
45. Satō, *Takano Chōei*, p. 141.
46. Satō, *Yōgakushi ronkō*, p. 177.

Chōei's accomplice, Eizō, was an outcaste (*hinin*) who worked along with a group of about thirty outcastes in the escort of prisoners and in various jobs in the prison. In the "wanted" posters distributed after Chōei's flight, Eizō was described as having been born in the province of Etchū and at the time of writing was about thirty-two or thirty-three years of age. He had been tattooed twice and had difficulty in extending both of his hands.[47]

This description deserves some explanation. There were two types of outcaste called *hinin*: those who had been born into that class; and those who had for some reason or other been demoted to it. There were many ways of becoming a *hinin*: for example, through a criminal act such as attempted double suicide, gambling, juvenile petty theft, or incest. During the Tenpō period, however, it was common for the *hiningashira*, those in charge of the compounds where *hinin* lived, to make a swoop on the poor and homeless in the vicinity and enter them on the register of outcastes. They were then given a home in a special compound and put under the control of the leader of the compound (*koyanushi*). However, many found it unbearable and ran away. This was a punishable offense, and if caught, a *hinin* would be tattooed from the left shoulder to a point about nine centimeters down the arm. Upon his second attempt, he would be tattooed on his left wrist. If he were caught a third time, he would be killed.[48] Eizō's attempts to run away are a strong indication that he was not a *hinin* by birth. Moreover, as a disabled person, he would have been susceptible to an "outcaste hunt." From the description that Eizō had twice been tattooed, we can learn that he had twice tried to run away and had been tattooed as a punishment.

Chōei presumably knew of the precariousness of Eizō's position when he chose him as his accomplice. Probably, Chōei also knew that, because he often came in and out of the prison to work, Eizō was not monitored closely by the prison guard. As someone who was probably not born an outcaste, Eizō was in some ways like

47. Takano Chōun, *Takano Chōei den*, pp. 27, 35.
48. Takayanagi, *Edo jidai hinin no seikatsu*, pp. 17–30, 88–90.

Chōei, a prisoner who desperately believed in the injustice of his condition. In finding for his accomplice another man who had nothing more to lose, Chōei's shrewdness is impressive.[49] At the same time, the relationship of these two men is worth considering. Probably it was built up over some time, and it seems to reflect a certain affinity that Chōei had with the underdog. Even in his earliest letters, Chōei appears to have been something of a victim of his own generosity in helping those in unfortunate circumstances.[50] Surely he would not have been able to tempt Eizō into so dangerous a plot by money alone.

Tragically, however, Eizō was to meet a grim fate. After the fire, it seems that at first his role in the escape was not fully realized, and that he was counted merely as one of the escapees. However, he was later captured and confessed that he had been paid by Chōei to set fire to the prison. He was indicted and executed in the fourth month of 1846.[51]

Chōei lived the remaining years of his life as a fugitive. At first, he appears to have lived off the money he had saved in prison. Thereafter, he relied on the protection of trusted friends, sympathetic daimyo, and his skills as a translator. There are several different accounts of his movements after the escape. What seems clear is that he traveled as far north as his native Mizusawa and Yonezawa before returning to Edo; and that from 1848 to 1849 he lived under the protection of Date Munenari of Uwajima domain on the island of Shikoku. Munenari was interested in using Chōei's translation skills in studying Western defense techniques. As knowledge of the Opium War spread, many daimyo became increasingly concerned about boosting their defenses; in this respect, Chōei was lucky that his skills were in demand. Almost all the translations completed after his escape from prison concern military science. Nevertheless, a fugitive, however useful, cannot complain about his meager wages, and, despite the stability of his posi-

---

49. I am indebted to Satō, *Yōgakushi ronkō*, p. 180, for this interpretation.
50. See Nakamura, "A Portrait of Takano Chōei."
51. Satō, *Takano Chōei*, p. 145.

tion, it seems to have been financially a difficult time for Chōei, who had a wife and children to support in Edo.[52]

In 1849, the news reached Chōei that his presence in Uwajima had been discovered. He fled immediately, traveling slowly to Edo via Hiroshima, Unomachi in Shikoku, and Nagoya. He was finally found by police at his home in Aoyama, Edo, on the thirtieth of the tenth month, 1850. He had moved there only three months previously with his wife and children, to practice medicine under the name of Zawa Sanpaku. Popular legend has it that he burnt his face with chemicals so as to disguise it. Some have described the move to Aoyama itself as a suicidal act,[53] and perhaps it was, for the area was home to members of the *hyakuningumi dōshin*, the type of police who found him.[54] The stress of living six years on the run, trying to eke out a living, and rumors that restrictions on the translation of Western books were to be introduced by the Bakufu, must have taken their toll. These restrictions were officially announced in the ninth month of 1850. Only books that had been inspected at Nagasaki were permitted to be bought and sold, and anyone dealing in or translating books other than these would be punished. Daimyo wishing to translate books about defense were required to first obtain permission and present a copy of the translation to the Bakufu when completed.[55] There is evidence that, shortly before Chōei died, he visited an acquaintance in Katori, leaving his two-volume dictionary and a translation of a military book in exchange for a loan of five *ryō*. As Satō suggests, two things can be read from this action: that Chōei was desperately in need of money, and that, with his last major translation completed, he had given up the idea of trying to live as a translator.[56] Perhaps his optimistic spirit had indeed at last been broken.

The precise circumstances surrounding Chōei's death are unclear. Some say he stabbed himself in the neck when confronted by

---

52. Ibid., p. 202.
53. Ibid., p. 216.
54. Satō, *Yōgakushi no kenkyū*, p. 500.
55. Satō, *Takano Chōei*, p. 209.
56. Ibid., pp. 212–13.

the guards, others suggest he was beaten to death. There was a trial held afterward, in which he was sentenced to death posthumously. His wife Yuki was forced into retirement. According to one writer, their daughter Moto was sold to a Yoshiwara brothel and died in a fire there after the great earthquake of 1855.[57] It is unknown what eventually became of Yuki or her two sons by Chōei, the second of whom was born in the year his father died.

Teachers and Students

By some accounts, Chōei is said to have been arrogant and competitive among his colleagues.[58] On the other hand, he seems to have been blessed with the ability to build up warm and trusting friendships. His students, in particular, were prepared to risk everything to hide and protect him after his escape from prison. The loyalty of Chōei's students is an extreme example of the teacher-pupil relationship in the Tokugawa period, for of course not every student was tested by his preparedness to protect a convicted criminal. Even so, there does seem to be a special element of trust in the teacher-student relationship of this period. As we shall see, this relationship had roots in a tradition of secrecy and had enormous implications for the exchange of knowledge at this time.

In Tokugawa Japan, there was no officially recognized system of medical training or qualification. Some teachers awarded their students certificates when they became independent, which no doubt carried some degree of weight, and some individual domains, such as Matsushiro domain in Shinano, introduced papers of accreditation in order to raise the standard of doctors,[59] but there was in general nothing to stop those with very little training from presenting themselves as medical practitioners. At the same time as there were doctors as well educated as Chōei, anyone who was capable of reading one or two medical books could make himself a doctor.[60]

---

57. Ōtsuki, "Takano Chōei gyōjō itsuwa," p. 396.
58. Ibid., p. 397.
59. Aoki, *Zaison rangaku no kenkyū*, p. 257.
60. Maruyama, *Gunma no ishi*, p. 24.

Similar to the case in eighteenth-century England, where the vast majority of medical practitioners were ordinary surgeons or apothecaries who learned by apprenticeship,[61] medical education in Tokugawa Japan was also usually undertaken in an apprenticeship or private school run by an established practitioner. Medical apprentices usually lived and worked with their teachers for a period of some seven to ten years, during which they progressed from running simple errands to reading the Chinese classics (or study of the Dutch language, in the case of Western medicine), and from there to mixing medicines and accompanying the practitioner on visits, and finally to studies of medical textbooks.[62] In the later stages of their training, apprentices would be allowed to represent the practitioner in his absence.[63] Evidence of this progression can be seen in Takahashi Keisaku's diary. His chief apprentice Gōsai began by helping around the farm and ended up attending Keisaku's patients in his own right.[64] There was a great deal of trust invested in this long and intense relationship, and medical practitioners and students alike needed to think carefully before committing themselves to it.

When Chōei first arrived in Edo and began to search for a suitable teacher, he did not yet seem to have understood the importance of this commitment. In a letter to his uncle in 1820, Chōei described how he approached one teacher, Toda, and made use of his accommodation, while fully intending to find someone else. Not surprisingly, Toda angrily threw him out when the truth was discovered:

Although I made various enquiries, there was not one place that would take us on . . . after consulting with Toda I gave him one month's board until another teacher could be found. As Toda seemed willing to put us up as we pleased, I went to consult with cousin Yōrin. We decided that we should move our baggage into Toda's house, as though we were to become his pupils. However, as I wanted to search for another teacher, I

---

61. Porter and Porter, *Patient's Progress*, pp. 19–20.
62. Maruyama, *Gunma no ishi*, p. 29.
63. Ono, *Edo no machiisha*, p. 233.
64. See p. 167.

suggested that Yōrin become Toda's pupil in my place, to which, much to my relief, he readily agreed. However, when the matter came to Toda's ears, he was furious.[65]

Connections and letters of introduction were all-important. Teachers often appear to have looked after young men from the same province as themselves. Toda Kensaku in the letter above, for example, was originally a native of Ichinoseki, quite near Chōei's birthplace of Mizusawa, and this may well have influenced his decision to give him lodgings. Chōei appears to have believed his father's connections to Sugita Genpaku would win him a place with his heir, Sugita Hakugen, but he was hindered because his adoptive father, Gensai, had not supplied him with suitable letters of introduction. Chōei goes on in the same letter of 1820 to explain how he eventually talked his way (somewhat untruthfully) into acceptance:

I had no other choice but to go immediately to Sugita-*sensei*[66] to whom I said, "Toda Kensaku is from the same region as I, so I met him and for the time being, upon his orders, became a boarder at his house. When I received a letter from home, I was intending to come in any case, but the letter has not yet arrived and as Toda is very poor at the moment, I hesitate to board there for a long time. If it could in some way be arranged, I hope very much you will have me," and so on. Sugita-*sensei* looked as though he thought it a great imposition, but he said that as my situation could not be helped, he would allow me to visit as a day student. I went to reason with him again but he seemed far from understanding.[67]

Chōei was disappointed in Hakugen's responses because, unlike a full apprentice, a day student had to find and pay for his own lodgings, rather than board with his teacher. Even when one had proper letters of introduction, the search for a teacher was not an easy task. Chōei's brother Tansai (who came to Edo at the same time) had to rely on the good offices of a man from Mizusawa to find him a place, after his letters of introduction had proved to be of no use.[68]

----

65. Takano Chōei Kinenkan, ed., *Takano Chōei no tegami*, pp. 8–9.
66. *Sensei* is a respectful term of address, meaning "teacher."
67. Takano Chōei Kinenkan, ed., *Takano Chōei no tegami*, pp. 10–11.
68. Ibid., pp. 12–13.

The importance of trust in the teacher-pupil relationship also manifested itself in other ways. Some apprentices were required to sign contracts when they graduated, promising that they would not divulge medical secrets learned in the practice to others.[69] Secrecy was vital to protect the interests of doctors in an open medical market where there was no minimum standard of qualification. The transmission of secret knowledge, not only regarding medicine, but also many other technologies, had been practiced by families and clans in Japan since ancient times. Families tried to keep a hereditary control on their professions by keeping knowledge within the family. Many doctors trained their sons as their medical apprentices. The secretive nature of medical training also helped to define the boundaries between various schools of medical thought. This tradition of secrecy was widely used in many private schools in the Tokugawa period[70] and was as important in schools attended by only a few students as in those in which there were hundreds. For example, in a certificate awarded by Hanaoka Seishū (1760–1835), there were many references to the secret teachings his student had received. Hanaoka had one of the largest schools in the country, with students numbering in the hundreds.[71] It has been suggested, however, that due to social changes, this closed system was beginning to break down by the middle of the Tokugawa period.[72] This change had important implications. As doctors were allowed more freedom to move about from teacher to teacher and to exchange medical ideas, it provided a social catalyst for developments in medical theory.[73] As will be discussed in the next chapter, the lecture series given by Takano Chōei in rural Nakanojō in 1833 is a significant example of the way that doctors were breaking out of these traditional patterns of secrecy.

Evidence in Chōei's letters that both he and his brother began to earn money from their medical activities while still undergoing

---

69. Maruyama, *Gunma no ishi*, p. 29.
70. Rubinger, *Private Academies of Tokugawa Japan*, pp. 155–57.
71. The certificate is quoted in Maruyama, *Gunma no ishi*, p. 32.
72. Rubinger, *Private Academies*, p. 157.
73. Johnston, "Jūhasseiki Nihon no igaku ni okeru kagaku kakumei," p. 11.

training attests to the idea that medicine could be freely practiced without qualification. After being accepted by Sugita Hakugen as a day student, Chōei lodged at the Kanzakiya, a pharmacy run by a friendly man from Mizusawa, and began to work at night to earn enough for his meals:

Well, it is said that having an artistic accomplishment can save one from ruin. I am at last making use of the massage that I learned previously in Higashiyama. When I go out every night, I can manage about four customers on a good night, about two hundred *mon*. . . .Using this money I buy my morning and evening meals, although it is not much, at a teahouse.[74]

As a medical apprentice, Chōei thus appears to have kept himself afloat by working as a masseur. Massage was traditionally associated with bone setting and with acupuncture. In the Tokugawa period, massage commonly became the work of blind people, especially under the influence of a man called Sugiyama Waichi (1613–94). Sugiyama developed a technique of using a special tube to help insert acupuncture needles. He eventually rose to fame, and after he successfully healed the shogun Tsunayoshi (1646–1709) of an illness in 1685, he received an official stipend. Under the auspices of the Bakufu, Sugiyama set up centers in many provinces where students were trained in his techniques. The blind masseurs formed guilds and had a licensing system. Despite their capacity to earn quite well, however, the status of masseurs and acupuncturists generally remained low, and higher-class doctors sometimes looked down upon the practice.[75] Nevertheless, it was not entirely unusual that Chōei should practice massage. First, he was not in a position to be choosy about his work. In addition, in the late Edo period, a new style of massage called Yoshida-*ryū* (style) was popularized, and massage performed by sighted practitioners flourished.

As early as 1822, when he was still only eighteen years old, Chōei wrote of treating patients on a journey to Nikkō. The fol-

---

74. Takano Chōei Kinenkan, ed., *Takano Chōei no tegami*, p. 12.
75. Fujikawa, *Nihon igakushi kōyo*, 1: 56–57, 138, 147–49. See also Casal, "Acupuncture, Cautery and Massage in Japan"; and Kokushi Daijiten Henshū Iinkai, ed., *Kokushi daijiten*, 1: 401.

lowing year, his brother Tansai fell gravely ill and died. Chōei was forced to neglect his studies and become responsible not only for his brother but also for his brother's patients.

Although we do not have anything much left over, Tansai has a few patients and I go about treating them. It is very worrying to go out and leave Tansai on his own, so I have asked a neighbor to look after him. By going out to work, I am able to make just enough to cover our meals, but have nothing in the way of savings.[76]

In 1825, Chōei made the long journey from Edo to Nagasaki to further his studies, as one of the privileged few to study with Siebold. There, he wrote of his studies:

The Dutch [*sic*] doctor with whom I am currently studying has an excellent reputation and the many students come from all over, so the school is at the height of prosperity. The Dutch doctor is extremely interested in medicinal plants and sometimes [we] go out to collect them. Also, we go out to treat the townspeople and so on; it is indeed most enjoyable.[77]

In Nagasaki, Chōei was able to support himself by making translations for wealthy Japanese residents and also for Siebold himself. In a letter to his adoptive father in 1827, Chōei wrote:

I have been doing translations from day to day for a man called Matsubara Kenboku, who pays for such things as my food supplies. A wealthy resident of Hagi, Chōshū, by the name of Kumagai Gorōzaemon is currently staying in Nagasaki, and since he has a long-standing interest in *rangaku* I have translated some materials on the theory of health care for him.[78] So little by little I have been receiving his support. Also, for Siebold, I have been translating some materials from Japanese into Dutch, which helps to cover various expenses. In any case, since coming here I have for the first time managed to escape hardship in having enough to eat, drink, and for miscellaneous expenses.[79]

---

76. Takano Chōei Kinenkan, ed., *Takano Chōei no tegami*, p. 24.
77. Ibid., p. 104.
78. Miyashita, "A Bibliography of the Dutch Medical Books Translated into Japanese," p. 21. This translation was called *Ransetsu yōjō roku* (Record of Dutch healthcare) and was a translation of a work by Hufeland, undertaken jointly with another of Siebold's students, Oka Kenkai.
79. Takano Chōei Kinenkan, ed., *Takano Chōei no tegami*, p. 106.

Matsubara Kenboku's real name was Yamada Taien (1756–1831). He was a doctor, and it appears that he had accumulated a large debt to Kanzakiya, the pharmacy where Chōei had lived in Edo. When the proprietor of Kanzakiya discovered that Yamada was living in Kyushu under the name of Matsubara Kenboku, and was working for the daimyo of Hirado, he generously instructed Chōei to go and collect the money from him and use it toward his studies. In the summer of 1826, Chōei set off for Hirado. When he arrived, Yamada unfortunately did not have the money to repay him, but he did have access to the large library of Dutch books belonging to the domain and arranged for Chōei to be able to read them. Before long, he was living at the Hirado domain quarters in Nagasaki, making translations for the daimyo.[80] In fact, his trip to the islands of Iki and Tsushima in early 1828 appears to have been an official one undertaken for the daimyo.[81] These favorable circumstances must have greatly assisted Chōei's work. Indeed, they may well have been the reason he did not accompany Siebold on his official journey with the Dutch to Edo in 1826. In a letter dated the tenth month of 1825, Chōei wrote to his adoptive father: "Although I was expecting to return to Edo next spring with the Dutch party, having nothing to show for coming all this way to Nagasaki, I would very much like to stay here next year and continue my studies. If I choose to do so, there are people here who are prepared to look after me; so I am trusting their judgment."[82]

From this time on, Chōei seems to have become increasingly scholarly, relying less on practical healing skills than on his linguistic and academic talents. This career path was to lead him in quite a different direction from ordinary doctors. Eventually, it was to lead him to his tragic downfall. At this juncture, it may be helpful to examine the many different types of medical practitioner in Tokugawa Japan, and what, indeed, an "ordinary doctor" was.

---

80. Satō, *Yōgakushi ronkō*, p. 152.
81. Satō, *Takano Chōei*, p. 46.
82. Takano Chōei Kinenkan, ed., *Takano Chōei no tegami*, pp. 101–2.

Schools and Identities

In most histories, medical practitioners are discussed in terms of their intellectual training or "school." The main schools of medicine in Tokugawa Japan are discussed briefly in the Introduction. This kind of approach tells us a great deal about the theories behind the therapeutics of the day, but little about how doctors went about their everyday lives, and whether this differed from school to school. On the other hand, medical schools seem to have formed an important part of how practitioners saw themselves and other doctors.

Chōei's sense of identity, for example, can be seen in a letter dated 1823, when he wrote: "This year, I hear there will be a re-registration of doctors. Even if I have to beg, I want to put my efforts into *rangaku*." The precise nature of this registration of doctors is unclear, but Chōei's loyalty to his subject is obvious.

What kind of relationship, then, did doctors from differing schools of thought have with one another? As noted above, the atmosphere of secrecy surrounding medical education did little to encourage harmonious relations. Western medicine in particular seems to have been viewed with a great deal of suspicion by some Japanese schools of Chinese medicine. It is well known that fear and jealousy of *rangaku* in its more political form was one of the reasons behind the *bansha no goku* oppression of 1839, in which Chōei was imprisoned. Writing in prison, Chōei described the situation:

Recently *rangaku* has greatly proliferated, with each branch of learning ranging from medicine as a matter of course, through to astronomy, geography, military strategy, and engineering, having its own *rangaku* school and specialist. . . . Moreover, because Western geographical studies shed light on things such as war and peace, the customs, human character, and rise and fall of all nations, recently various great scholars have turned their attention to *rangaku* and taken it up rather than Confucianism. As a result, there are other people who are full of hatred and jealousy [toward these converts].[83]

---

83. Takano Chōei, "Wasuregatami," pp. 173–74.

The repression of the *bansha no goku* was followed by a dark period for Western learning. Medicine actually fared better than other disciplines, for it alone was exempted from a general ban on Western learning in 1840, but it did not escape when this climate of oppression culminated in 1849 with an outlawing of all forms of *ranpō* medicine except surgery and ophthalmology. According to Bowers, the ban was never strictly enforced,[84] but it nevertheless remained in place until 1858. The powerful and conservative Taki family, with its strong connections to the Bakufu, appears to have been influential in the suppression of Western medicine during this period.[85]

At the same time, it is important to recognize that not all doctors trained in Chinese medicine were antagonistic to Western medicine. Hanaoka Seishū, who emphasized Chinese theory and Western techniques, is a fine example of this. It has been noted how many doctors from the *koihō* school seem to have moved quite easily into Western medicine, because of a similar emphasis on practical rather than speculative methods, and an understanding of the body based on scientific anatomy rather than Confucian philosophy.[86] Chōei's friends from Kōzuke, who were in their thirties and forties before they moved from *koihō* to *ranpō* medicine, exemplify this trend.

Despite differences in theoretical orientation, approaches to diagnosis and therapeutics were quite similar. There was, moreover, an increasing trend toward empirical observation. According to Confucian approaches to medicine, the purpose of diagnosis was to identify the nature of the imbalance in the body that was causing illness. In particular, it was important to determine such factors as whether the problem was yin or yang, cold or warm in nature, and whether the symptoms were external or internal. This diagnosis was usually achieved by four methods: observation (visible symptoms and general appearance), listening (breathing and coughing), questioning (patient history), and palpation (especially pulse tak-

---

84. Bowers, *Western Medical Pioneers*, p. 143.
85. Hattori, *Edo jidai igakushi no kenkyū*, p. 14.
86. Johnston, "Jūhasseiki Nihon no igaku ni okeru kagaku kakumei," p. 15.

ing). The *koihō* school doctors tried to introduce new methods of examination in addition to these and placed a special emphasis on stomach palpation.[87] Yoshimasu Tōdō developed a theory of "all diseases, one poison," which meant that doctors could just treat the area that was affected by poison, rather than trying to discern the cause of the illness. Stomach palpation was conducted to find the location of the poison. He thought that the poison should be treated by giving poison (medicine) and tended to prescribe stronger medicines than the *goseiha* doctors.[88] Tōdō's son Nangai, however, later advised against diagnosing purely on the basis of symptoms and went about revising the "all diseases, one poison" theory. He warned that it was possible for the same disease to cause different symptoms or the same symptoms to be caused by different diseases. His theory was based on the idea that poison was caused by blockages in either *ki* (fundamental energy), blood, or water in the body.[89] Regardless of the practitioner's medical orientation, the patient could expect to be treated by a combination of herbal (and sometimes Western) medicine, acupuncture, moxibustion, massage, respiratory therapy, and remedial exercises.

Similarly, apart from the intricacies of diagnosis, the everyday life of medical practitioners seems to have differed less according to intellectual school than according to popularity and status. Status was, however, to some extent related to the type of medicine practiced. Doctors of internal medicine, or *hondō*, were considered to be true doctors and had the highest status. Other types of practitioners, such as surgeons and acupuncturists, were considered to be technicians, rather than theorists or scholars.[90] As we have seen, there was also a certain degree of hierarchy among the medical schools, to the frustration of proponents of Western medicine. The appointment of the Taki family as hereditary directors of the Bakufu's official medical school underlined the political power of conservative Confucian medicine.

---

87. Fujikawa, *Nihon igakushi kōyō*, 1: 186.
88. Lock, *East Asian Medicine*, pp. 54–55.
89. Fujikawa, *Nihon igakushi kōyō*, 1: 168–69.
90. Johnston, "Jūhasseiki Nihon no igaku ni okeru kagaku kakumei," pp. 9–10.

Livelihoods

The lack of formal standards of qualification in the Tokugawa medical market meant that there was an enormous range of ability among medical practitioners. It is helpful, then, to classify medical practitioners according to their status or social role. There were two basic types: those with official, salaried appointments and those without. Salaried doctors included those who served the court, the Bakufu, and daimyo governments. Some of these positions were hereditary, but there were also opportunities for talented doctors to obtain official posts.

In the Bakufu, there were more than ten ranks of salaried doctors. The highest-ranking position was largely an administrative one and was hereditary, filled by members of two families. Next in rank were those directly responsible for the care of the shogun's everyday health and medical oversight of the women's quarters. These doctors were called *okuishi* and were appointed by merit. There were usually about sixteen *okuishi* in total, divided into specialties of internal medicine, surgery, acupuncture, ophthalmology, and dentistry. Although the value of Western surgery had been recognized in the appointment of Katsuragawa Hoshū (1751–1809) as an *okuishi* surgeon, the power of conservative medicine within Bakufu circles in the nineteenth century meant that it was not until 1858 that *ranpō* physicians, such as Totsuka Seikai (1799–1876) and Itō Genboku (1800–71), were finally appointed to this high-ranking position.[91] Interestingly, it was the inability of the established *okuishi* to heal the shogun Iesada's (1824–58) illness that seems to have provided the impetus for this appointment.[92] The ban on Western medicine enacted in 1849 was also lifted concurrently.

Lower-ranking official doctors were responsible for other groups within the castle. There were opportunities, too, for promotion by merit by attracting the attention of daimyo leaders. Daimyo tended to base their medical bureaus on the Bakufu sys-

---

91. Hattori, *Edo jidai igakushi no kenkyū*, p. 769.
92. Ibid., pp. 709–10.

tem, although this naturally differed slightly from domain to domain.[93] Daimyo appear to have been generally less conservative about the promotion of doctors from different intellectual schools or from the lower classes. For example, Itō Genboku, who was of humble origin, was recognized by the Saga domain as early as the 1830s, well before he finally became an *okuishi* in the Bakufu.[94]

Official doctors who were able to live off their medical salaries seem to have existed even in ancient Japan.[95] By the first half of the nineteenth century, the *okuishi* Taki Anshuku is said to have received as much as 2,000 *ryō* per year.[96] Most doctors, on the other hand, earned much less, and it has been suggested that official doctors were actually rewarded quite poorly compared to other kinds of official appointments.[97] As an example of the salary of a domain doctor, Tsuboi Shinryō received about 30 *ryō* per annum when he was appointed an official doctor to Echizen domain in 1853.[98] Perhaps the situation in Tokugawa Japan was similar to that in England, where poorly paid public appointments were sought for their prestige and the likelihood of attracting patients to private practice.[99] A salaried position did at least give the medical practitioner some guaranteed income as well as the opportunity to enhance his reputation.

In contrast to salaried doctors, private practitioners, who in towns were known as *machiisha* (town doctors), battled to make a living in a highly competitive market. They were hampered by a traditional tendency to see medicine as an act of charity rather than as a livelihood. Rich salaried doctors could afford such acts of philanthropy, but ordinary practitioners needed to make their living.

Some doctors needed to overcome a personal reluctance to receive money for medical treatment, and they did this by adopting

---

93. Fujikawa, *Isha no fūzoku, meishin*, pp. 33–34.
94. Goodman, *Japan: The Dutch Experience*, pp. 177–78.
95. Fujikawa, *Isha no fūzoku, meishin*, p. 47.
96. Nakajima, *Byōki Nihonshi*, p. 291.
97. Fujikawa, *Isha no fūzoku, meishin*, p. 51.
98. Miyachi, *Bakumatsu ishinki no bunka to jōhō*, p. 193.
99. See Anne Digby, *Making a Medical Living*.

certain methods. For example, the amount paid was sometimes left
to the patient to decide.[100] It was also sometimes paid in kind.
Humorous poems testify to the way the amount of rice one paid
the doctor could be subject to the scrutiny of one's peers in the
waiting room.[101] Payment was generally seen to be for the medicines dispensed, not for the medical skills provided by the practitioner.[102] This was a problem particularly at the higher end of the
social scale. In England, it was not until the mid-nineteenth century that trained physicians came to be paid for their services.[103]
There, the custom among the upper classes was to bill yearly, and
the problem of nonpayment was such that sometimes practitioners
found it helpful to employ debt collectors on commission to collect their fees by installments.[104] In Japan, too, since medical fees
were usually only collected twice a year, at New Year and the Bon
festival in the middle of the year, the collection of fees was a des-
perate problem for practitioners. Chōei complained of this problem in a letter to his father in 1823:

This Bon festival season, the collection of fees was extremely difficult and
I managed to collect about four *ryō*, not even a half of what I anticipated. . . . When I added up the monthly expenses, even though I econo-
mized, they amounted to more than one *ryō* and two *bu*. I made the
treatment for syphilis payable in cash; so I had for the time being just
enough to make do, but I still owed a little for the cost of medicines from
Kanzakiya. With the money that you sent last time, I was able to pay off
everything, and I do not owe anything to anyone.[105]

Chōei's letter also gives a good indication of how much he
earned as a young medical student. Far from the 2,000 *ryō* earned
by the shogun's doctors, he scraped by on four *ryō*, perhaps eight, if
he collected fees twice a year. What did this amount mean in real
terms? In the late Tokugawa period, one *ryō* could generally buy

---

100. Fujikawa, *Isha no fūzoku, meishin*, p. 49.
101. Ono, *Edo no machiisha*, p. 50.
102. Fujikawa, *Isha no fūzoku, meishin*, p. 48.
103. Digby, *Making a Medical Living*, p. 37.
104. Ibid., p. 158.
105. Takano Chōei Kinenkan, ed., *Takano Chōei no tegami*, pp. 35–36.

about one *koku* of rice, which was about enough to feed an adult for a year, and a male wage laborer could earn around three *ryō* per year over and above his food and clothing.[106] In individual cases in the 1840s cited by Hanley, a tenant farmer earned twelve *ryō* per year, and a carpenter in Kyoto earned double this.[107] This tends to confirm Fujikawa Yū's theory that the status of unsalaried doctors in the Tokugawa period was roughly equivalent to that of peasants.[108] Unlike a wage laborer or tenant farmer, however, Chōei presumably had to buy his own food and pay his school fees from his earnings. As can be seen from the letter above, he also had the burden of purchasing medicines for his patients, from whom he had no guarantee of payment. Even taking into account the fact that he does not seem to have been very good at managing his finances, it is not difficult to see why he still depended on his adoptive father for financial support.

As we have seen, during the 1830s Chōei was assisted financially by three doctors from rural Kōzuke. These men, by contrast, appear to have been quite well off, but they were supported by secondary occupations: Fukuda Sōtei ran an inn; Takahashi Keisaku was a farmer; and Yanagida Teizō had a large inheritance. It is difficult to determine what proportion of their wealth came from medical activities. The medical fees that Takahashi Keisaku recorded in his diary range from as little as ten *hiki* (about a hundred copper *mon*) to as much as one *ryō*, but the majority of payments were in *hiki*.[109] This suggests that he adjusted his fees according to the wealth of his patients, or that they simply paid him whatever they could.

When a doctor gained enough experience, he could "open his gate" and begin to take students. Teaching was a very useful way of making extra income. Fees in private schools were usually paid in the form of an entrance fee, followed by fees for the teacher's services, to be paid regularly at festival times.[110] Similarly, in Kōzuke,

---

106. Smith, *The Agrarian Origins of Modern Japan*, p. 125.
107. Hanley, *Everyday Things In Premodern Japan*, p. 20.
108. Fujikawa, *Isha no fūzoku, meishin*, p. 31.
109. Kanai, *Takahashi Keisaku nikki*, pp. 581–82.
110. Rubinger, *Private Academies*, pp. 70–71.

Takahashi Keisaku's pupils frequently brought a gift of wine upon entering the arrangement, as well as at the end of the year.[111] The fees at schools of Western learning in Edo appear to have been very expensive, much more so than at Confucian or National Learning (*kokugaku*) schools. One scholar suggests a figure of around five *ryō* per year for the school of Tsuboi Shindō (1795–1848), one of the leading scholars of Western learning in Edo.[112] Shindō is said to have made as much as 600 to 700 *ryō* per year.[113] In a society that was becoming increasingly entrepreneurial, success was no longer dependent on official appointment. Personality did play an important role, and it has been suggested that Chōei's inability to flatter his patients was a factor in his failure to become a popular doctor.[114] One might also surmise that he was more interested in his own research and translation than in visiting patients or, indeed, in making money.

Types of Doctors

It has already been suggested that doctors of internal medicine distanced themselves from other kinds of medical practitioners. Just as in England, where (to a certain point) medical practitioners were divided into physicians, surgeons, and apothecaries, there were several types of practitioner in Tokugawa Japan. There was no official system of training or registration in Japan, but the hierarchy of status appears to have been quite similar. Doctors of internal medicine (the physicians of England, by comparison) were seen to be mainstream. Judging from the diary of Takahashi Keisaku, they treated a variety of disorders, including fevers, colds, digestive problems, sexually transmitted diseases, eye problems, and some skin problems.

---

111. For example, on 1864.1.25, when five new students entered Keisaku's school, they brought five *shō* of *sake* (presumably one each) and three small dishes. Wine was the most common end-of-year gift Keisaku received.

112. Quoted in Rubinger, *Private Academies*, p. 121.

113. Quoted in ibid., p. 135.

114. Sugiura Minpei, *Kazan to Chōei*, p. 105.

Surgeons, who had prospered in wartime, found in Tokugawa peacetime that their work was mainly confined to treating injuries, boils, and sexually transmitted diseases. They tended to be looked down upon by other doctors because of their association with knives and cutting, needles, and moxibustion.[115] Satirical poems suggest that they set up their practices in rough neighborhoods so that they might profit from the injuries resulting from quarrels that went on there. One poem pointed out rather cruelly that a doctor who treated hemorrhoids "ate off the bottoms of others."[116] But this was not the entire picture. Hanaoka Seishū, mentioned above, mixed his surgery with Chinese internal medicine and was tremendously successful. Takahashi Keisaku, as a country doctor, was more or less obliged to take on surgical cases. Farming was a dangerous occupation, and he was called to many accidents that required stitches. Far from finding this degrading, he seems to have taken a special interest in these cases, recording them in unusual detail in his diary.[117]

Other doctors specialized in eye problems or women's health. So-called women's doctors were in many cases actually abortionists. The abortionists appear to have flourished despite a ban on the practice introduced in the Shōhō years (1644–48). There were both male and female women's doctors, who developed a custom of hanging long curtains at the entrance to their practices for privacy and built several entrances, so that it was easy for people to come and go quietly. Pompe van Meerdervoort, a Dutch doctor at Nagasaki, observed in his diary from the years 1857–63:

In Nagasaki, there were two old women who were notorious because of their way of practicing abortus by means of a lance which they were able to handle quite well. To these and similar individuals, people in Japan sometimes go for help, and I must say that it is specifically the wealthier ones, those who would be quite able to support their children, who most frequently do this. Another woman achieved the same effect with live mercury; she did not have such a large practice because the results were

---

115. Fujikawa, *Nihon igakushi kōyō*, 1: 138.
116. Ono, *Edo no machiisha*, pp. 61–62, 83–85.
117. See p. 144.

not always successful. As soon as I had sufficient proof of the actual existence of these crimes, I discussed this with the authorities in charge, but they found my complaints exaggerated. It is true that murder was outlawed in the country, but then the victim would be alive first, and an unborn fruit was not considered to be a living individual as yet. It belonged to the mother, they said, as part of her body, and she was free to do what she wanted with that body. I did not succeed in bringing about any improvement in this state of affairs, and both ill-famed women still carry on a thriving practice as "famous abortionists."[118]

Although Pompe's account gives no indication of it, abortionists could be looked down upon. They were seen to carry the spiritual weight of the work they did, and if they vacated their premises, others were reluctant to move in, at least until proper purification prayers had been performed:

> *Chūjō no ato, akidana de yayashibashi*
> After the abortionist, the shop stays vacant for a while.
>
> *Chūjō no ato, yagitō ni nen wo ire*
> After the abortionist, take care with the house-blessing.[119]

Abortionists were able to charge high fees due to the delicate nature of their business. Some of them even gained an evil reputation for lending money at high rates. Other poems refer to how abortionists were able to build grand storehouses with their ill-gotten gains, without ever a patient to be seen.[120]

Childbirth was usually assisted by female relatives or, increasingly, by midwives, who were known as *toriagebaba* (literally, old-women-deliverers). Pompe noted in his diary how in wealthier families, an experienced woman would be employed to stay with the family her entire life.[121] The midwife usually had no special training, other than her many years of experience. Even her apprentices were said to start at age fifty or more. Although little is known about how she was paid, a midwife's work was treated

---

118. Wittermans and Bowers, eds., *Doctor on Desima*, p. 39.
119. Ono, *Edo no machiisha*, p. 110.
120. Ibid., pp. 100–111, 142–44.
121. Wittermans and Bowers, eds., *Doctor on Desima*, p. 41.

seriously. For example, midwives had special permission to cut across daimyo parade trains and would not be questioned by local town guards. Her work was not confined to the birth itself; she usually attended every night for the first seven days to bathe the newborn baby. Indeed, Pompe found that the parturient woman was usually the victim of too much attention, rather than too little:

She is not allowed a moment's rest until the whole act of delivery is completely finished. Every moment she is shifted from one position to another, now higher, then lower; on the back, then turned on the side. . . . Japanese midwives have the idea that "rest" after the delivery is particularly harmful, and they do not even allow the woman in childbed the sleep which contributes so much to restore the forces spent during delivery. The reasons are superstitious in origin, although I have never heard a clear statement about it.[122]

If the birth was complicated, the midwife sometimes called in a male doctor to assist.[123] This is evidenced by the fact that Takahashi Keisaku assisted at several births in Kōzuke.[124] Pompe, however, complained of the lack of scientific knowledge of obstetrics among Japanese doctors. He made only one exception: Siebold's daughter, Ine, in Nagasaki. When he saw her serving as an obstetrician for European women, he found that "she really was most satisfactory."[125]

Quack doctors were known as *yabui* (bush doctors) or *takenoko-isha* (bamboo shoot doctors). Presumably, "bamboo shoot" doctors were young, green, and inexperienced. The origin of the expression "bush doctor" is less clear. One suggestion for the name is that this type of doctor could not afford to buy his own medicines and went into the bushes to collect them himself.[126] *Yabui* were the subject of many humorous poems. They blundered about in their shabby clothes, killing patient after patient, better known for their fast talking than their medical skills. Some of them associated with

---

122. Ibid., p. 42.
123. Ono, *Edo no machiisha*, pp. 245–67.
124. See p. 145.
125. Wittermans and Bowers, eds., *Doctor on Desima*, p. 42.
126. Ono, *Edo no machiisha*, p. 179.

the professional jesters (*taikomochi*) of the pleasure quarters in order to make a living on the side, and others, taking advantage of their wide circles of acquaintance, were employed as matchmakers.[127] Although these poems probably contain an element of truth, it is worth remembering that not all alternative practitioners were frauds and that for mainstream doctors, denunciation of "quackery" was the only defense they had against it. As Dorothy and Roy Porter have argued in the context of eighteenth-century England, quack medicines might taste better or sometimes even work better than regular medicines, as well as being cheaper. In such medically uncertain times, patients were often willing to try anything, seeking the advice of both regular and irregular practitioners.[128] Both trained and untrained doctors at times found themselves the object of distrust and ridicule.

Doctors and Status

The struggle for status often manifests itself in appearances. In England, it has been suggested that patients were inclined to put their faith in social criteria such as the personal connections, grooming, or tact of physicians, because the rudimentary state of medical knowledge did not allow a great deal of public confidence in their healing abilities.[129] Physicians, therefore, had to earn the trust of their patients on an individual basis.[130]

In Tokugawa Japan, physicians adopted a particular style of dress in order to set themselves apart from ordinary commoners. They did this within the confines of a dress code based on class distinctions, and the trend became increasingly pronounced over the course of the period. Originally, doctors shaved their heads and dressed much as priests did, in a kimono (*kosode*) with a short coat (*jittoku*) over the top. This was the formal dress of doctors, paint-

---

127. Ibid., pp. 175–213.
128. Porter and Porter, *Patient's Progress*, pp. 106–7.
129. Peterson, *The Medical Profession in Mid-Victorian London*, p. 130.
130. Porter and Porter, *Patient's Progress*, p. 58.

ers, poets, and priests.[131] Gotō Konzan of the *koihō* school was influential when he rebelled against this practice by pulling his hair back in a ponytail, wearing a divided skirt (*hakama*), and a special coat (*hōekihō*).[132] The *awase* was a coat adapted from the European cape. Most people wore it short, but samurai, wealthy commoners, priests, and doctors took to wearing a longer style.[133] Doctors were also famous for their *haori*, another kind of coat. Unlike samurai, who wore the *haori* more formally with a divided skirt, doctors simply wore it over their kimono. For this reason, the *haori* became something of a trademark of the doctor.[134] Thus, although prevented from dressing as samurai, commoner doctors distinguished themselves in various ways from ordinary folk.

By the nineteenth century, doctors were being criticized for their luxurious habits. Here is what one writer had to say:

Because their fees are too generous, doctors these days neglect their studies and grow increasingly extravagant. Their clothes are exquisitely beautiful and their houses have proper entrances, studies, and every other amenity. Even their servants exercise their authority. At home, they live in a most noisy and ill-mannered fashion and eat only the best food and drink. Because they do not understand the deeper principles of medicine, they are unkind. While ostentatiously behaving as if they were the epitome of a good doctor, they deceive people. Doctors with official posts and those with something of a reputation are especially proud, and they ride in palanquins even when visiting patients. Their palanquin bearers and other attendants behave like samurai. In addition, there are some attendants, who work for the recent new kind of popular doctor, who try to make themselves look busy and rush around the streets creating more fuss than a samurai's passing, troubling people when their paths cross. Sometimes they start a quarrel, and if anyone should happen to touch the medicine box, it immediately comes to blows. They take an aggressive stance, saying that the medicine chest is an important tool for the medical way. When these attendants go to visit a patient, it is customary for them to demand money for their "lunch," sometimes 50 *hiki*, sometimes 100, or

---

131. Tanida and Koike, *Nihon fukushokushi*, p. 104.
132. Fujikawa, *Isha no fūzoku, meishin*, p. 55.
133. Tanida and Koike, *Nihon fukushokushi*, p. 125.
134. Fujikawa, *Isha no fūzoku, meishin*, p. 41.

200 *hiki*. This is enough to buy a half, or one or two bags of rice. Even though there are just four or five of them, this is more than enough lunch money to feed eight or nine people.[135]

The situation was such that at last the Bakufu government was forced to issue an edict in 1841 prohibiting doctors' attendants from demanding money for *sake* or lunchboxes when accompanying the doctor on medical visits.[136] These documents provide an interesting indication of the medical practitioner's rise in importance (or at the very least, self-importance) in the late Edo period. By association, even his attendants appear to have felt that they could put on airs.

There were various methods popular doctors could employ to attract more patients. One well-known strategy was to keep a large number of people in the waiting room in order to create the appearance of a flourishing practice. Even when this was not the case, it took time to grind and dispense medicines. Many humorous poems depict such a scenario:

> *Dokaochi no senu yō ni isha hito wo tame.*
> The doctor hoards people, to avoid a slump.
>
> *Shibaraku mataselamae chōgō no jisetsu*
> Mixing medicine: make them wait a little.[137]

The bored patients slowly began to show their frustration:

> *Ryūkō isha genkan ni taenu ōakubi.*
> At the door of the popular doctor, endless, huge yawns.[138]

If the poems are to be believed, some patients appear to have entertained themselves with all sorts of antics: fighting over sunny spots, tidying their beards, chain-smoking, gambling, even writing obscene graffiti on the unfortunate doctor's wall.

Not only did patients waiting for their medicines become restless, they also became hungry:

---

135. From *Fūzokukenbunshū*, vol. 2, quoted in Fujikawa, *Isha no fūzoku, meishin*, p. 42.

136. Fujikawa, *Isha no fūzoku, meishin*, pp. 39–43.

137. Quoted in Ono, *Edo no machiisha*, p. 36.

138. Quoted in ibid., p. 38.

Ōzei ni hidarugarasete chōgō shi
Mixing medicine makes the masses hungry.[139]

Kusuritori kanzō kuite shikarareru
Waiting for medicine: scolded for eating the licorice.[140]

It should be remembered that only popular doctors could afford to treat their patients this way. As an example of life at the other end of the social scale, there are poems poking fun at quack doctors borrowing their shabby long coats, getting motion sickness on unfamiliar palanquin rides, and bringing in their bumpkin attendants from the country.[141]

Something should perhaps be said about the sheer number of humorous poems concerning doctors. It suggests a remarkable fascination with them, in all their various categories. The desire to poke fun at doctors may well have come about through a general uncertainty and a touch of jealousy about their new place in society. As Porter and Porter have suggested with regard to the situation in England, it was natural for people to distrust doctors when increasingly they were putting themselves in their hands.[142] Furthermore, they argued that the "growing affluence and airs of the rank-and-file of the profession excited astonishment and envy."[143] Significantly, there were complaints about the pretensions of physicians in England, hurtling around the streets in their chariots, just as we have seen in the Japanese example above.[144]

Although they usually go hand in hand, wealth is not always commensurate with status. By the late Tokugawa period, the traditional class distinctions of warrior, farmer, artisan, and merchant had become blurred. Many wealthy commoners were better off than lower-ranking samurai. If Chōei's students from Kōzuke are any indication, the life of wealthy regional farmer-physicians, for example, appears to have been quite comfortable, and within the

------

139. Quoted in ibid., p. 47.
140. Quoted in ibid., p. 48.
141. Ibid., pp. 181–86.
142. Porter and Porter, *Patient's Progress*, p. 57.
143. Ibid., p. 126.
144. Ibid., p. 124.

confines of the village they enjoyed an elite status. Quite apart from the fact that there was probably a genuine need for local physicians and a great deal of moral satisfaction to be gained from helping one's own community, it is not unreasonable to think that men such as these were quite content to be big fish in a small pond.

For those who desired it, however, there were opportunities for outstanding scholars, regardless of hereditary rank, to rise to advisory positions. Takano Chōei is a fine example of this ambition, for although he was of middle-ranking warrior class by birth, he chose to reject the stipend and comforts of family succession for an ambitious scholastic career. There is a suggestion, too, in Fukuda Sōtei's poems, that he had a frustrated desire for greater things.

In his essay on "Center and Periphery," Edward Shils described society as having a less geographical than social center, dominated by the value system created by elites.[145] He argued that most of the masses in premodern societies did not notice their alienation from such a "center." There were, however, some more "sensitive or intelligent" persons, who became acutely aware of their position on the outside and often gained access to the center by becoming schoolteachers, priests, or administrators.[146] Although it is uncertain whether Shil's vision of society can be applied across boundaries of space and time, this idea does find some echoes in Totman's idea of the "savant" in Tokugawa Japan.

Totman used the word "savant" to refer to the career paths of physicians, teachers, or scholar-advisors.[147] A scholarly career was an attractive way in which masterless samurai (rōnin) could make a living, because it had a fluid status not specifically defined by the hereditary system of "samurai-peasant-artisan-merchant." This was particularly true of the careers of scholar-physicians. Physicians who were engaged by daimyo or the Bakufu as advisors could gain a great deal of wealth and prestige, normally available only to those who had been born to it.

---

145. Shils, "Center and Periphery," pp. 93–95.
146. Ibid., p. 106.
147. Totman, *Early Modern Japan*, pp. 163–66, 186, 349.

As Totman has indicated, there was also considerable respect for the scholarly tradition of Chinese medicine, for it involved the study not only of practical therapies but also of classical Confucian texts. A physician might well turn to a teaching career and evolve into a scholarly advisor. Although the early savants were mainly masterless samurai, in the later Edo period, scholarly careers were increasingly important as a means for wealthy commoners to improve their status. Totman has given the example of Itō Jinsai (1627–1705) as a fine example of a scholarly commoner.

Although Takano Chōei was robbed of the opportunity to reach the heights to which he aspired, in many ways he seems to epitomize the career of the savant. A rōnin of his own volition, he professed that he would rather take his chances on an interesting scholarly career than be safely tied to rural obscurity in Mizusawa. It is here, of course, that Chōei differed from his friends in rural Kōzuke, because, although they continued to have important social and intellectual links to Edo (and thus in Shils's scheme of things, maintained access to the central value system of the elite), they seemed content, or at the very least resigned, to building their careers in their rural homeland.

Medical practitioners in the counties of England have been described as "marginal men," that is, men who moved in more than one social world but belonged to none.[148] They were "marginal" both in the sense of belonging to an occupational group that had not yet established its place in society, and because they lived in the counties, rather than in fashionable London. Upwardly mobile doctors such as these had a particular need to appeal to the community for their status, and they did so through activities such as work on committees, in local literary societies, public donations, and the dissemination of medical information through public lectures. Many parallels may be drawn between the ways in which physicians attempted to attain respect and wealth in nineteenth-century rural England and the social and academic activities engaged in by Takahashi Keisaku in rural Kōzuke.

---

148. Inkster, "Marginal Men: Aspects of the Social Role of the Medical Community in Sheffield 1790–1850," p. 128.

A similar comparison may be drawn in Australia, where it was easy for elite physicians, who had the ability to draw on traditional class mechanisms, to become involved in public affairs and active as community leaders.[149] So, in Japan, too, the nineteenth century saw the rise of wealthy farmer-physicians in rural areas, who made use of the affinity between public affairs and medicine. Aoki has suggested that it was easy for powerful farmers and village officials to become doctors because the conditions under which they operated were in many ways complementary.[150] In their positions of power, it was easy for such local officials to gain access to medical information. If notices arrived from official domain doctors, it was the village officials who would have to read and distribute the information among the villagers, and in such cases, some kind of medical knowledge was often helpful. Village officials served as distributors for official medical supplies and were therefore in a good position to receive information about medicines. They also maintained useful connections with official doctors and private medical suppliers. Through their administration of mountains and fields, local officials had knowledge of the medicinal plants that grew there. Wealthy villagers were able to pay for medical services and drugs themselves. They could afford to spend money on medical education and books and possessed the time and necessary skills to read them. Their social status meant that they associated with warriors, official physicians, and other wealthy commoners.

Medicine also had a role to play in the maintenance of the local political system. A village official who gave gratis medical treatments, whether officially supplied or of a personal nature, would help to consolidate his position in the community. In many cases, public health measures were the responsibility of village officials. Thus, powerful locals would be able to gain respect by becoming medical practitioners, and similarly, those who were already physicians were looked up to as local elites.

The importance of the local doctor has been illustrated by Aoki, who introduced documents that show how villagers without the

---

149. Willis, *Medical Dominance*, p. 45.

150. This section is based on Aoki, *Zaison rangaku no kenkyū*, pp. 257–75; and Aoki, "Sōmō no rangaku," pp. 219–68.

services of a physician attracted them to their communities by drawing up contracts and paying them out of village funds.[151] In one example, the villagers supplied a house for the doctor and his family, paid for his medical expenses in the event that he became sick, and even contracted to pay his funeral expenses if necessary. A contract was often for three years, but if the doctor was well liked in the community, the agreement could be extended. The conditions would depend somewhat on the financial status of the village. A physician in a rural community was also desirable because he often had a role to play as a teacher, not only of medicine, but also of local children in a *terakoya* school. The popularity of these schools, which provided a basic education, reflects an increasing awareness of the value of literacy among commoners. Some doctors were hired specifically to be local teachers. Aoki's examples come from Shinano (Nagano prefecture), but among the Kōzuke physicians of this study too, both Fukuda Sōtei and Takahashi Keisaku appear to have taught medicine. In addition, Keisaku was employed in his later years as a *terakoya* teacher. A document from 1869 records that he had as many as 85 pupils over the years.[152]

These examples demonstrate that doctors such as Takano Chōei and the Kōzuke physicians, who were by no means elite physicians in the sense of being domain doctors or serving the shogunal family, were able to command a certain amount of respect within their communities. On the one hand, by virtue of his scholarly abilities, Chōei was accepted into a circle of quite high-ranking scholars and officials in Edo. The Kōzuke physicians, on the other, were part of a local elite. They were by no means poor, although it is difficult to know what percentage of their earnings came from medical activities. Takahashi Keisaku and Yanagida Teizō belonged to families who traditionally served as village officials; Keisaku himself became headman in 1857. The Kōzuke physicians may be seen to typify a new kind of rural doctor who emerged from within the level of the local elite in the early part of the nineteenth century.

151. Aoki, *Zaison rangaku no kenkyū*, pp. 171–80.
152. Kanai, *Takahashi Keisaku nikki*, p. 565.

CHAPTER 2

The Kōzuke Physicians:
Rangaku *in the*
Countryside

Nestled among the mountains of provincial Kōzuke (present-day Gunma prefecture), the villages around Nakanojō might seem an unlikely setting for lively scholastic activity. Nevertheless, in the 1830s, the region was the picturesque backdrop to a number of exchanges between Takano Chōei and a network of country doctors. Chōei shared his knowledge of Western medicine with his provincial friends through visits, lectures, letters, and, eventually, two collaborative publications. Their activities provide an excellent example of the way that rural doctors were actively seeking knowledge, including Western knowledge, even in remote, mountainous areas of Japan well before the Meiji period.

The first part of this chapter explores the significance of Nakanojō as a geographical backdrop to medical networking. It paints a picture of nineteenth-century rural society in order to see how the rise of medicine and networks fitted in with contemporary economic and social developments. The second part of the chapter introduces the lives of the Kōzuke physicians, their medical community, and the nature of their connections to Chōei. This leads into a final section that examines the growing network of *ranpō* doctors beyond the borders of Kōzuke.

A Place to Practice

A contemporary journey from Tokyo to Nakanojō on the Agatsuma train line provides a scenic introduction to the area's geography. The great metropolis of Tokyo fades slowly to flat fields
dotted with buildings, interspersed again with the built-up areas of
Takasaki and Maebashi. The level Kantō plain is left abruptly at
Shibukawa, as the train swings to the northwest and begins to
climb. Following the course of the Agatsuma River as it flows
from the west down into the Tonegawa at Shibukawa, the line
passes through Nakanojō before terminating in the mountains at
Ōmae. The entire journey now takes less than three hours. In the
Edo period, it usually required four days.[1]

Nakanojō is situated in the center of the Nakanojō plain, a
mountain plain that stretches along the middle reaches of the
Agatsuma River about 350 meters above sea level. The plain is surrounded by mountains on all sides: Takeyama in the north, Yaku-
shigatake in the west, Harunasan in the south, and Jūnigatake and
Onokoyama in the east. The mountains and the bubbling rivers
that flow into the Agatsuma are spectacularly beautiful. Indeed,
Nakanojō and nearby Sawatari thermal springs, about ten kilome-
ters to the northwest, are not unworthy of their place on one of
Japan's "romantic roads" for tourists. Although Nakanojō now
administratively incorporates several villages, such as Sawatari,
which are dotted along the local rivers, these villages originally had
quite separate identities.

As a natural link between the mountain and farming villages
further beyond in the north and west and towns on the Kantō
plain, Nakanojō was ideally situated for economic exchange. There
is some evidence that, as a result of increasing economic activity,
the region was already beginning to take on such a role even before
the Edo period. Thereafter, Nakanojō continued to develop as a
market town, which marketed locally some rice that came through
from Echigo on its way to Edo, and acted as a post station, which
provided horses and other transportation facilities.[2]

---

1. Kanai, "Rangaku to waga Nakanojōmachi," p. 1112.
2. Koike, *Edo jidai no Nakanojōmachi*, pp. 4–7.

Nakanojō's success as a market town was partly due to a lack of rice in the local region.[3] Although the center of Nakanojō's economy was essentially agriculture, the nature of the land and climate allowed only a small quantity of poor-quality rice to be grown. The main crops were barley, wheat, millet, buckwheat, red beans, white radishes, and other vegetables, grown in dry fields. In addition to these, Takahashi Keisaku planted rape seed, burdock, corn, cucumber, and eggplant, as well as cash crops such as mulberry and tobacco. Men were able to supplement their incomes by ropemaking and woodcutting. Women wove cloth and participated in sericulture.[4] Paper, oil, tofu, and many other daily necessities could be bought at the market. Local breweries sold rice wine, and there were cloth dyers and pharmacies in town.

Nearby Sawatari thermal springs appear to have had even fewer agricultural opportunities. Apart from some dry field farming, charcoal making, lacquer work, and a little silk farming were carried out. Interestingly, a number of guns were permitted in the village, and hunting was customary.[5] Sawatari appears to have had its heyday in the early part of the nineteenth century, when it began to develop as a resort. Important to both the development of Nakanojō as a post station and Sawatari as a thermal springs resort was good access to the Tokugawa transportation network.

Roads for transport and communication were essential to the political functioning of the Tokugawa state. Initially, they were used to move armies and officials and to send messages. Later the roads became important for daimyo paying their respects in the capital and for the transportation of tax rice.[6] The Tokugawa shogunate extended its control over the transportation network by nationalizing five important highways and eight auxiliary roads, equipping them at regular intervals with a system of post stations to supply horses, porters, and accommodation to official travelers. To assist with the economic burden placed on the town, a post sta-

---

3. Ibid., p. 6.
4. Kadokawa Nihon chimei daijiten hensan iinkai, ed., *Nihon chimei daijiten*, 10: 691.
5. Karasawa, *Agatsuma shichō*, p. 146.
6. Vaporis, *Breaking Barriers*, pp. 17–18.

tion was granted tax exemptions and had a salaried manager. Daimyo employed a similar system of roads, post stations, and official documents in their own domains.[7]

Nakanojō and Sawatari thermal springs did not lie directly on national highways, but they did have important connections to them. Nakanojō lay on the Nitta (Numata) road, which already was an important road in medieval times. This road connected Nakanojō with Nakayama post station, which lay on the north-south national highway, the Mikunikaidō, and Numata further east. In the west, the road passed through Naganohara and the barrier station at Ōse, before crossing the border into Shinshū (Nagano prefecture). Nakanojō was also connected to the north by the Mikunikaidō Wakiōkan, an important supplementary road running from Nakanojō through Sugawa to Nagai post station near the Echigo border.[8] As a post station, Nakanojō had a role to play in supplying transportation services. Most goods were moved in and out of the town by pack horse, and many residents were involved in this business, either full time or in the agricultural off-season.[9] The main road was interspersed at regular intervals with inns and teahouses to provide for the needs of travelers.[10]

The main road from Nakanojō to Sawatari thermal springs formed part of the Kusatsudō, an important road running from the nearby resort town of Kusatsu, through Sawatari, Nakanojō, the springs at Ikaho, and finally to Edo.[11] This road was opened in the Edo period and prompted a great increase in the number of travelers from Edo.[12] Sawatari was also connected to Nakanojō's rival market town of Haramachi by a road that connected with the barrier station of Ōto, on the Shinshūkaidō. This way was not as steep as the Kusatsudō and was, in economic terms, an important road for Sawatari. Incidentally, according to Kanai, this is the road

---

7. Ibid., pp. 22–26.
8. Based on entries and maps in *Nihon chimei daijiten*.
9. Koike, *Edo jidai no Nakanojōmachi*, p. 7.
10. Kanai, *Takahashi Keisaku nikki*, p. 206.
11. Kanai, "Fukuda Kōsai no rangaku no michi to Agatsuma rangaku," p. 30.
12. Karasawa, *Agatsuma shichō*, p. 114.

by which Fukuda Sōtei sent his mail to Edo and by which he received his medicines from Takasaki.[13]

In terms of administration, excluding a brief period in which it formed part of Numata domain, the land around Nakanojō remained essentially directly in the hands of the Bakufu throughout the Edo period. At times the area was administered by a government intendant (*daikan*), whereas in later periods it was divided up into two *hatamoto* domains.[14] The province of Kōzuke as a whole was important to the Tokugawa government as a defense against the Tōhoku and Kansai areas, and many chief retainers were placed there. That the administration of Nakanojō remained under central rule therefore can be thought of as a reflection of its geographical role as a gateway to the Kantō plain. It was also significant for the Kōzuke physicians, in that they were in close contact with administrators who often had business in the capital.

In addition to these geographical factors, there were a number of broader social and economic changes that assisted the rise of commercial medicine in rural areas. Such trends became increasingly pronounced in the second half of the Tokugawa period.

The Popularization of Culture: Travel and Amusements

In early nineteenth-century Japan there was a "flowering of material and artistic culture in the great urban centers."[15] It was a period characterized by the commodification of culture, its incorporation into daily life, and the rise of the information age. Some of the activities that typify the culture of the early nineteenth century include a publishing and reading boom, visible in the proliferation of booksellers and lending libraries; training in light artistic accomplishments, particularly among young girls; a passion for street theater and festivals and places of amusement; and tourism and pil-

---

13. Kanai, "Fukuda Kōsai no rangaku no michi to Agatsuma rangaku," p. 31.

14. *Hatamoto* (sometimes translated as "bannermen") were shogunal retainers of middling rank.

15. Jansen, "Japan in the Early Nineteenth Century," p. 71.

grimage.[16] These kinds of activities were enjoyed particularly, although not exclusively, by commoners, and not only in urban areas but increasingly in rural ones too.

The commercialization of the economy, especially in rural areas in this period, increased the need for travel, and hence for facilities such as well-maintained roads and post stations. With improved communications and increasing travel, there were many opportunities for cultural interaction. In areas outside the great cities, castle towns, post stations, and thermal springs resorts were often the focus of commercial and cultural activity. Along with important shrines and temples, thermal springs were extremely popular travel destinations in the nineteenth century for those with sufficient financial resources. Patients usually made their journey to the thermal springs on foot and stayed for quite long periods of time.[17] Despite the traditional image of the Edo period as a time of immobility, travel restrictions, within Japan at least, do not seem to have been as severe in reality as they were on paper, and travel on medical and religious grounds was readily approved.[18]

Nakanojō and Sawatari thermal springs, too, were able to prosper during the Bunka and Bunsei years (1804–30). Evidence of the lure of Nakanojō can be seen in the way people floated in from Echigo and Shinshū in search of work. Men usually found work in breweries or as sweet-makers, while women worked in food stalls, in inns, or as waitresses.[19] Perhaps they also worked as prostitutes, which were common in inns and thermal springs resorts. Apart from workers such as these, there was a general flow of travelers and tourists through the area, from whom, as we shall see, Fukuda Sōtei was able to benefit. One reflection of this is that in a report he made about the people he treated, there were many more people from Edo than from Nakanojō.[20]

---

16. Takeuchi, "Shomin bunka no naka no Edo," pp. 7–8, 54.

17. Watanabe, *Edo no onnatachi no yuami*, p. 199.

18. Jansen, "Japan in the Early Nineteenth Century," p. 64; Vaporis, *Breaking Barriers*, p. 5.

19. Koike, *Edo jidai no Nakanojōmachi*, p. 11.

20. Kanai, "Fukuda Kōsai no rangaku no michi to Agatsuma rangaku," p. 36.

Thermal springs have had an important role as places of healing throughout Japanese history. Judging from archaeological evidence, it is likely that humans, like the animals they hunted, used thermal springs for bathing from prehistoric times.[21] This is also true of places in England like Bath, where it is believed early humans were attracted to the good hunting around the hot springs.[22] The area around Nakanojō and the springs at Sawatari too have revealed archaeological remains dating from the Jōmon period.[23] From early times, springs were associated with healing miracles and were called *kami no yu*, or "divine baths."[24] They were dedicated to holy men, saints, or figures such as *yakushi nyorai*, the Buddhist "physician of souls."[25] Springs were used by warriors to heal their wounds, to the extent that in the Warring States period, the famous general Takeda Shingen (1521–73) banned civilians, nobles and commoners alike, from using the springs at Kusatsu so that they could be used exclusively by his warriors.[26]

Thermal springs were often used to provide relief from diseases that affected the skin, such as syphilis, scabies, and hemorrhoids. They were also said to be helpful in the treatment of rheumatism and lameness. Keisaku's daughter-in-law Kise, for example, made a journey to the springs at Ikaho in 1868 because she was suffering from severe pain in her left shoulder. She returned home after about six days, having found no relief.[27] Other women made journeys to hot springs if they were having difficulty in conceiving.[28]

Due to the varying qualities of their waters, most thermal springs gained a reputation for the treatment of specific diseases. Kusatsu was popular for the treatment of syphilis. This disease, for which doctors could do little apart from drastic mercury treatments, was frighteningly common in Tokugawa times. At Sawatari

---

21. Taketa, *Furo to yu no koborebanashi*, pp. 2–3.
22. Cuncliffe, *The City of Bath*, p. 2.
23. 10,000–300 BCE.
24. Grilli and Levy, *Pleasures of the Japanese Bath*, p. 109.
25. Taketa, *Furo to yu no koborebanashi*, p. 6.
26. Karasawa, *Agatsuma shichō*, p. 125.
27. Kanai, *Takahashi Keisaku nikki*, pp. 364–65 (1868; pp. 4, 9–15).
28. Watanabe, *Edo no onnatachi no yuami*, p. 206.

too, Fukuda Sōtei's father (referred to here as Sōtei IV) made a medicine for syphilis that sold well.[29] Sawatari was most famous for skin complaints. It was particularly popular as a stopping place for patients on their way home from Kusatsu to Edo. Not only was it en route, but the waters at Sawatari were also perfect for soothing skin roughened by the acidic water at Kusatsu. In this way, Sawatari was able to benefit directly from the success of Kusatsu as a resort town.

In Kusatsu, a popular destination for Edo dwellers, people normally stayed at least ten days, which was known as "one round." Some patients stayed for as long as five rounds.[30] During their visits, patients would usually rent a small room and cook for themselves. Basic cooking equipment was borrowed from the proprietor of the inn, and other amenities could be bought from merchants in the town. There were also teahouses, archery ranges, lending libraries, and so on to cater to the visitors. Many merchants were attracted from out of town, bringing their wares by horse or ox.[31] The influx of visitors thus helped to make thermal springs resorts important economic centers.

As the town of Sawatari began to prosper, Fukuda Sōtei, as his ancestors had before him, was able to combine successfully the roles of physician and innkeeper. Sōtei's ancestors are believed to have settled in Sawatari and worked as physician-innkeepers from the Kyōhō period (1716–36). From the Tenmei period (1781–89) on, there was an increasing number of visitors coming to the area, and many of them liked having a physician in the inn where they stayed. Sōtei IV prospered so well that in 1803, neighboring innkeepers filed a lawsuit against him.[32] The advantages that Sōtei IV's medical practice gave him were a source of great jealousy among the other innkeepers.

---

29. Kanai, "Fukuda Kōsai no rangaku no michi to Agatsuma rangaku," p. 34.
30. Gunma Ken Shi Hensan Iinkai, ed., *Gunma ken shi*, Tsūshihen 6, p. 265.
31. Ibid., pp. 265–67.
32. See Karasawa, *Agatsuma shichō*, pp. 158–67.

Pharmacies and the Circulation of Medicines

It has already been noted that Sawatari could not rely heavily upon its agriculture. In addition to the business of a thermal springs resort, the collection of medicinal herbs appears to have been an economic sideline. A merchant by the name of Arai Iuemon in Haramachi, for example, sent local game and medicines to Takasaki and Edo.[33] Indeed, all over the country, hunters, itinerant priests, and ascetics who lived in the mountains had a role to play in collecting bear gall, monkey brains, fox liver, and the like for medicinal purposes.[34] In Shinshū, which, like Kōzuke, was mountainous, medicines have been documented as an important part of the pack-horse trade.[35] The increasing commercialization and circulation of medicines in the Edo period were part of more general economic changes such as urbanization, rural commercialization, better transportation, and rising living standards for many groups of people. In villages, people "were gradually able to buy goods that had been previously available only in urban centers or to purchase items that had formerly been made in the household."[36]

Traditionally, most ordinary people were unable to pay a physician for medical treatment. They relied on prayer and folk remedies based on herbs they could collect themselves. For example, many people presented wooden tablets at temples illustrated with, or cut in the shape of, the part of the body they hoped to heal. Tablets painted with eyes were very common, which suggests that eye diseases were a problem in the Edo period.[37] Home remedies included, for example, an infusion of dried earthworms for fever, a type of Chinese bamboo (nandina) for stomach pains, and balloon flower root for coughs.[38] Increasingly, however, people relied on commercial preparations too. Originally, it was physicians who

---

33. Kanai, "Fukuda Kōsai no rangaku no michi to Agatsuma rangaku," p. 31.

34. Sugiyama, *Kusuri no shakaishi*, p. 166.

35. Aoki, *Zaison rangaku no kenkyū*, p. 169.

36. Hanley, "Tokugawa Society: Material Culture, Standard of Living, and Life-Styles," p. 696.

37. Tatsukawa, *Edo yamai no sōshi*, p. 375.

38. Sugiyama, *Kusuri no shakaishi*, p. 112.

collected or bought crude drugs from pharmacists and mixed them appropriately. In the Edo period, however, especially from the end of the seventeenth century, some drug merchants began to mix and sell their own preparations.[39] Handbooks for household medicines also became popular. Niwa Seihaku and Hayashi Ryōteki, for example, wrote a book, *Fukyū ruihō* (Treatments for dissemination), in 1729, in which they selected medicines easily obtainable in mountains and fields, in order to help people in remote villages who had poor access to pharmaceuticals.[40] As Yoshioka has pointed out, household manuals also gave people clues as to how to go about making their own medicines, both for sale and for private use.[41]

Not only drug merchants, but also physicians, warriors, temples, perfumers, and peddlers sold medicines. Drugstores tended to be confined to cities and towns, but peddlers took medicines all over the country.[42] Peddlers from Toyama used a system whereby they left their medicines with customers and came back later to collect money for those used and replace them if necessary. People could use only what they needed and pay for it later.[43] Commercial medicines were thus within the reach of most people. Some merchants advertised their medicines quite aggressively. Santō Kyōden (1761–1816), a popular writer who supported himself by running a drugstore, unashamedly made reference to his medicines in his literature, not merely in the form of advertisements but in the stories themselves. Another clever merchant by the name of Matsuura Shichibei (born 1782), who had a shop on the Nakasendō highway, lent umbrellas painted with his advertisements to travelers.[44]

Some drug merchants and temples handed down secret recipes from generation to generation, in the same way that physicians were careful to guard their family secrets. The mystery in which these medicines were shrouded often worked as a selling point.

---

39. Yoshioka, *Edo no kigusuriya*, p. 101.
40. Ibid., p. 35.
41. Ibid., p. 40.
42. Ibid., pp. 61–65.
43. Sugiyama, *Kusuri no shakaishi*, p. 165.
44. Amano, *Kusuri bunka ōrai*, p. 86.

Medicines developed by priests or temples, for example, although they were actually based on Chinese medical theories, were associated with magical religious properties and were very popular.[45] One such medicine, called *kintaien*, was sold at stalls in temple grounds where tourists and pleasure seekers gathered.[46]

Quite a large proportion of commercial medicines claimed to be cure-alls. This perhaps fulfilled a psychological need for reassurance on the part of customers who were trying to treat themselves.[47] This was also surely part of the success of medicines like *kintaien*. Thus the druggist played an important role for those who used self-medication rather than go to the trouble and expense of visiting a medical practitioner.

Pharmacies were quite numerous in post stations, where they could attract the custom of travelers passing through. In the Naka-nojō region, there were four pharmacies in the village of Isemachi alone. As we have seen, Fukuda Sōtei seems to have bought medicines from Takasaki, also an important post station and political center. Umenoki village, a post station on the Tōkaidō highway near Kusatsu (Shiga prefecture), became very famous for a medicine for stomach pains called *wachūsan*. Engelbert Kaempfer, who passed through there on a journey to Edo with the Dutch mission, gave a detailed description of the medicine and its sale:

The houses of Menoke (Umenoki) are scattered along the highway, and the village consists of several parts. It is famous for a powdered medicine called *wachūsan*, which was discovered here and cannot be produced anywhere else. This is taken as a remedy for a number of illnesses, but especially the local colic, and consists of putchuk (one of the foreign, bitter costus roots) and various local roots and bitter herbs growing in the surrounding mountains. They are ground to powder together with the costus (after all the ingredients have been dried and cut into rough pieces) and sold in three separate stalls and houses located at some distance from each other. On our return journey we saw that the grindstone is turned by four men the way our mustard seed mills are operated. The remaining work is carried out by two women, who gather up the powder and carry it into the warehouse. There it is wrapped into four-cornered pieces of

45. Ibid., pp. 60–72.
46. Takeuchi, "Shomin bunka no naka no Edo," p. 39.
47. Yoshioka, *Edo no kigusuriya*, p. 73.

paper, each side the width of four fingers, on which the name, strength, and dosage have been printed in red and black letters. Each portion of powder weighs a little over two drams and is taken one to three times with warm water depending upon the person and the illness. In these houses the same herbs are also steeped in fresh water and served like common tea to those who care for it. The inventor was a pious, poor man who lived in the settlement of Tebara. He claimed that the deity Yakushi (the local Apollo and patron of medicine) appeared to him one night in a dream, showing him these herbs in the mountains and ordering him to prepare them for the use of his sick fellow citizens. This claim benefited the medicine and its sales greatly, and in a short time he rose from poverty to position and wealth.[48]

This description provides a fine example of how such popular medicines were sold, and the potential wealth that they could bring to their inventors. Although Kaempfer mentioned only three stalls in Umenoki village, another author recorded that there were as many as 56 pharmacies there.[49] It was not only merchants and pharmacists but doctors, too, who made use of commercial medicines. Keisaku and his pharmacist friend, Koitabashi, made a medicine in 1872 that they called *dokushogan* (reading pills). Perhaps they were inspired to this by the commercial success many years earlier of Santō Kyōden, the writer mentioned above for his medical puffery. A medicine of the same name was one of his best-selling preparations. It was claimed to strengthen the spirit, assist with forgetfulness, colic, and general ill health, and was especially recommended for travelers and those in poor health, and during the hottest part of summer.[50] Similarly, an advertisement for Yanagida Teizō's practice mentioned a special eye medicine,[51] and as we have seen, Fukuda Sōtei IV sold a medicine for syphilis.

The rise of commercial medicine in late Tokugawa Japan is remarkably similar to the situation in England (particularly during the eighteenth century).[52] There, too, a culture of self-healing was

---

48. Kaempfer, *Kaempfer's Japan Tokugawa Culture Observed*, p. 328.

49. Amano, *Kusuri bunka ōrai*, p. 46.

50. Yoshioka, *Edo no kigusuriya*, p. 106.

51. A reproduction appears in Kanai, *Takano Chōei to Agatsuma*, p. 23.

52. This discussion is based on the information in Porter and Porter, *Patient's Progress*.

reinforced by medical consumerism. Doctors were not shy about self-publicity, and their puffery in newspapers and popular literature was akin to Santō Kyōden's stories. Just as Keisaku and his friends developed commercial medicines, doctors in England too were happy to put their names to nostrums. Porter and Porter argued that the freedom of capitalist relations in England, in combination with a tradition of independence, Protestantism, and Enlightenment individualism, contributed to the formation of this type of medical culture, which was absent in other European countries such as France.[53] A comparative analysis of this argument in the Japanese context is well beyond the scope of the present work, but that such a similar medical culture existed in Tokugawa Japan is certainly worthy of further investigation.

The Lectures of 1833

It was against this background of commercial and social developments that Chōei held a series of medical lectures in Nakanojō from the twenty-third of the seventh month until the twenty-fifth of the eighth month, 1833. They took place at the country villa of Yanagida Teizō, a wealthy Kōzuke physician, and were attended by a small group of interested locals. In addition to the host Teizō, present at the lectures were a pharmacist called Negishi Shūzō; three physicians, Mochizuki Shunsai (1802–45), Takahashi Keisaku, and Endō Yōrin (who was Chōei's cousin, living elsewhere in Kōzuke at the time); and a man by the name of Ichimata Junsai.

Details of Chōei's lectures and the names of the attendees were taken down in careful notes by Keisaku. Later, he lent these notes to his teacher of Chinese medicine, Itō Chūtai (Rokuri) (1778–1838), who copied them and left them for historians to discover, years later, in his storehouse in Nagano.[54]

Chōei based the lectures on his book *Fundamentals of Western Medicine*, which had been published just one year previously, in 1832. Significantly, it was this group of Kōzuke physicians that had

---

53. Ibid., p. 209.
54. The notes are reproduced, with a short introduction, in Aoki, "Itō Chūtai hisshya 'Takano shi sōbyōron.'"

given him financial backing for the work. It is therefore probable that the lectures were a way for Chōei to express his appreciation for their support.

Judging from their content, the lectures were by no means intended for a wider audience. In addition to the material based on his book, Chōei discussed the treatment of specific diseases and made a detailed theoretical exposition on the general theory of disease. In this, he explained that in the West there were two theories of disease: one that treated diseases as single entities, and one that explained the reasons behind all diseases. Following the ideas of G. W. C. Consbruch (1764–1837), he argued for a general theory of disease, in which illness occurred as the body's natural reaction against some kind of threat (usually the result of neglectful health practices). He preferred this theory to those arguing for imbalances in the body, pointing out how the eye produces water to flush out dust, and the skin produces pus to fight against a splinter. He went on to define a disease nosology based on symptoms, signs, and causes. He noted that there were some traditional classifications in the Chinese *Shōkanron*, such as the three stages of yin and yang, but criticized this work for making no mention of causes.[55]

This lecture series is of enormous historical significance, for it means that Chōei was delivering the latest in Western medicine from his recently published book to ordinary physicians and pharmacists in provincial Japan. Most of these local doctors had trained in Chinese not Western medicine. Modest and somewhat exclusive though the audience was, it gives an indication of a blossoming professional identity among the provincial physicians.

In the late Tokugawa period, it was quite common for Edo-based authors, artists, and poets to make tours of the countryside, giving lessons, lectures, and recruiting students, in order to raise funds.[56] Chōei, who, as we know, was always short of cash, would appear to have been no exception. Yet there is some evidence to suggest that his relationship with this group of doctors in rural Kōzuke evolved into something far more significant than merely a business arrangement based on financial need.

---

55. Ibid.
56. Howell, "Social Disorder and Moral Reform in Late Tokugawa Japan," p. 14.

Takano Chōei and the Kōzuke Physicians

As we have seen in the preceding chapters, Fukuda Sōtei, Yanagida Teizō, and Takahashi Keisaku were three physicians who lived in villages around Nakanojō. During the 1830s, when they became pupils of Western-style medicine, the three men built up a close association with Chōei. The famous *rangaku* scholar had many students during his lifetime, and the fact that he taught them is nothing remarkable in itself. Nevertheless, their relationship is worth considering for several reasons.

As we have already seen, the rural physicians became his patrons as well as his students, and helped to finance his important publications. They also assisted in inspiring and editing Chōei's works on famine. These works were precipitated by a visit Chōei made to Kōzuke in 1836. According to *Treatise on Two Things for the Relief of Famine*, which was the first of the collaborative documents, Sōtei gave Chōei some buckwheat, and Teizō gave him a potato; through their discussion, they interested him in these crops as a preventative measure against famine. Not only did the pair assist in editing the work, but they also gave it their financial support. On the other hand, Keisaku, who studied in Chōei's school in Edo, assisted Chōei in compiling *Methods of Avoiding Epidemic Diseases* from one of his previous works. The contributions of all three are properly acknowledged by Chōei in the works themselves. This, along with the fact that the Kōzuke physicians were roughly the same age as their teacher or only slightly older than he, suggests that their relationship may well have been quite collegial.

Fukuda Sōtei (Kōsai) was the oldest of the Kōzuke physicians, and it is he who is said to have been the initiator of the relationship with Chōei. There is, however, some confusion as to how it all began. The most common theory is that he invited Chōei to come to Kōzuke, most probably around 1831, the time when Sōtei, already in his early forties and a physician of considerable reputation, began to study the Dutch language.

Sōtei was born at Sawatari thermal springs, as the eldest son of a physician, in 1791. He had two elder sisters and a younger brother. It was customary for the head of the family to take the name of

Sōtei, and this Sōtei was already the fifth generation. After completing preliminary schooling with a Confucian scholar by the name of Maruyama Hakuhō in Nakanojō, Sōtei was sent at the age of seventeen to Edo, where he studied the Confucian classics under Ichikawa Beian (1779–1858). Beian's father, Ichikawa Kansai (1749–1820), was a highly distinguished poet, a fact which may have influenced Sōtei's poetic inclinations.[57] Following this, he studied medicine under Ninomiya Dōtei, a physician of the *koihō* school. It was not until the age of thirty, that, shortly before his father's death, he returned to Sawatari to take over the family practice.

Perhaps assisted by the long history of his family as local physicians in the area, Sōtei became an extremely successful rural physician. He was able to maintain secondary practices in Haramachi and as far away as Takasaki.[58] Of his personal life little is known, although Sōtei does appear to have been married twice. His second marriage took place in 1836, to a woman called Nobuko. It was she who bore Sōtei his two children, Haruko and Bundō.

According to the inscription on Sōtei's burial monument, his interest in Western medicine was sparked when, frustrated with his inability to heal certain ailments, he was impressed by a translation of a Dutch medical book and began to experiment with the treatments described therein.[59] Kanai Kōsaku has suggested that the book may have been J. A. van de Water's pharmaceutical treatise, a book listed on the ledger of the pharmacy Sōtei patronized. However, since a translation of this work was not published until 1856,[60] this is highly unlikely. Keisaku made a copy of this work too, but this was not until 1860.

Concrete evidence of Chōei's first visit to Nakanojō is lacking and must be pieced together from accounts on the memorial tablets of Sōtei and Keisaku. If we are to believe these, Chōei first came to Nakanojō at the invitation of Sōtei, probably in 1831. Perhaps the visit was largely a social one, giving Sōtei the opportunity to meet Chōei and affording the scholar the opportunity to relax

57. Kanai, "Fukuda Kōsai no rangaku no michi to Agatsuma rangaku," p. 35.
58. Kanai, "Rangaku to waga Nakanojōmachi," p. 1121.
59. Kanai, "Fukuda Kōsai no rangaku no michi to Agatsuma rangaku," p. 37.
60. Nichiran Gakkai, ed., *Yōgakushi jiten*, p. 785.

in the waters of Sawatari thermal springs. Kanai has suggested that Sōtei's student, Takahashi Gentan, as well as Keisaku, were probably present at this first meeting. It is also likely that Chōei brought with him at this time chapters of the Dutch text that Sōtei proceeded to study by correspondence. The first 47 chapters of this text, which was a copy of a book on surgery by David von Geshez, were both copied and translated in Chōei's hand. Later chapters of the work were copied in Chōei's hand but translated in Sōtei's, giving an indication of his progress. The encouraging manner in which Chōei answered his pupil's queries remains documented in Sōtei's books. For example, Chōei praised one of Sōtei's translations, writing, "This chapter is very clear, with no mistakes at all." In another chapter, Sōtei wrote, "I cannot understand this chapter," to which Chōei replied that he could not understand it very well either.[61]

Despite Chōei's patient teaching, learning Dutch was not an easy task, especially with such limited resources. When Chōei made a third visit to Kōzuke in the eighth month of 1836, Sōtei recorded the occasion in his diary.[62] In the same entry, he also wrote down a proverb in Dutch, which translates roughly as "Drops of water make a stone hollow, not by their force, but because they fall so many times upon it." Usually, this is interpreted as Chōei's response to the frustrations expressed by Sōtei at the difficulties of learning Dutch.[63] In the same entry Sōtei noted down instructions for preparing a medicine that Chōei brought with him, along with the names of several of his teacher's associates in Edo.

In return for Chōei's lessons, Sōtei helped Chōei financially, in particular with the publication of his first major work, *Seisetsu igen sūyō* (Fundamentals of Western medicine). At the time of Chōei's visit in 1836, Sōtei's diary states: "Takano Zuikō came. Lent him *delie kopan* to have *Sūyō* carved for printing." *Delie kopan* is probably a corruption of the Dutch for "three *koban*," which were pieces of

61. Kanai, "Rangaku to waga Nakanojōmachi," pp. 1119–21.
62. Nakanojōmachishi Hensan Iinkai, ed., *Nakanojōmachishi shiryōhen*, p. 968. All further quotations from Sōtei's diary are from this source.
63. Kanai, "Fukuda Kōsai no rangaku no michi to Agatsuma rangaku," p. 38.

gold used in the Edo period.[64] As noted in the previous chapter, only the first part of *Fundamentals of Western Medicine* was originally published in 1832. This *Sūyō* therefore may have been one of the other parts, which had circulated in manuscript form, or, as Kanai suggested, the second volume.

The following letter was written by Chōei to Sōtei in 1838. It was a plea for financial aid to help with the reconstruction of his house after it was all but destroyed by fire:

It has not been long since I moved house, and in principle I should have been able to pay off my old debt by the coming seventh month. After the seventh month I was also looking forward to being able to pay back the money I borrowed last year. I am extremely perplexed to have had this stroke of bad luck. Accordingly, I ask you again even though I have not yet returned the money I borrowed last year. I have spoken of the matter of the timber and asked for your help. I assure you that you will not be out of pocket. As I said in the last letter, please help me just for a short while by sending the timber. I will pay you immediately it arrives.[65]

It was not only Sōtei who came to Chōei's assistance in this time of need. The Kōzuke group's efforts appear to have been coordinated by Negishi Kenbei, the local intendant (*daikan*). Evidence for this can be found in a letter thought to have been written by Kenbei to Mochizuki Shunsai, a doctor from Nakanojō who studied with Chōei in Edo and attended the lectures in 1833. In the letter, Kenbei asked Shunsai to inform his teacher that Sōtei would contribute 260 planks of cedar, Teizō 60 posts, and that he and his relative Shūzō (the pharmacist) would buy 100 pales (which were somewhat expensive).[66] Even if Chōei did intend to repay the loan as he claimed, their generosity and level of cooperation is remarkable.

Of Sōtei's personal character, it is said that he had a generous nature, and that he often treated poor patients free of charge, even going so far as to give them money for their journey home.[67] It

---

64. Kanai, "Rangaku to waga Nakanojōmachi," p. 1129.

65. Takano Chōun, *Takano Chōei den*, pp. 324–25. Maruyama Kiyoyasu quotes a section of this letter as being addressed to Yanagida Teizō. I have decided to follow Takano Chōun, who quotes the entire letter as being addressed to Sōtei.

66. Kanai, "Takano Chōei monka Nakanojōmachi Mochizuki Shunsai no hizō monjo o haiken shite," p. 21.

67. Maruyama, *Gunma no ishi*, p. 144.

would be easy to assume that such generosity, and also that displayed toward Chōei, meant that he had plenty of money to spare. This, however, does not appear to have been the case. Kanai demonstrates how, when his father died, Sōtei was left with many debts to families in neighboring villages, which, despite his booming practice, he struggled to pay off.[68]

In the third month of 1836, Sōtei made a resolution in his diary. In it, he promised to determine the duties of each day at daybreak, see patients until lunchtime, read and write poetry in the afternoon, and drink only two cups of wine with an evening meal of barley and vegetables. In an addition dated the seventh of the fifth month, Sōtei promised to give up the two cups of wine as well, the result of some gall pain brought on by the extended celebrations accompanying his second marriage. So sad and sorry did this make him that on the following eighth day, he chided himself for having made no progress in his studies and not perfected his skills, despite his 46 years, and having brought his illness upon himself through wine and women. We can suspect from this that Sōtei was cruelly self-disciplined. The doctor's dissatisfaction with his achievements also seems to be reflected in the following poems.

> The clergy in black and laity in white
> One after another, they visit.
> Medical diagnosis is already in decline;
> In our land, heroes can be counted on a few fingers.
> Sadness buried in my *sake* cup, I smile alone.

> The wind over Snake River billows and sighs heroically;
> A frosty wind dapples the peak of Mt. Haruna with color.
> A forty-year-old man, yet to gain a reputation;
> As my hair grows white, I shed secret tears.

> A precious sword, buried for an eternity in a box;
> Thick with dust, there has been no way to draw out its shine.
> No one yet knows its amazing value;
> Its rainbow like brilliance unrevealed, I cry alone in pain.[69]

---

68. Kanai, "Fukuda Kōsai no rangaku no michi to Agatsuma rangaku," p. 40.
69. Quoted in Kanai, "Fukuda Kōsai no rangaku no michi to Agatsuma rangaku," pp. 40–41.

Perhaps Sōtei regretted the lateness with which he had turned to Western studies, or perhaps he felt the limitations of his career as a provincial physician, especially after having lived such a long time in the capital. In any case, shortly before he died of a cerebral hemorrhage in 1840, the year after Chōei was arrested, he appears to have been a frustrated man. The inscription on his gravestone, said to have been written by his student Takahashi Gentan, records that he shortened his own life through his devotion to study and helping others.[70] Sōtei's son, Bundō, was as yet unborn when his father died. Sōtei was succeeded in his medical practice at first by a nephew, but Bundō eventually followed in his footsteps as the seventh-generation Sōtei.

Not far from Sawatari thermal springs, in the village of Isemachi (present-day Nakanojō), lived Yanagida Teizō, host of the 1833 lecture series. He too was a physician with a long family history of medical practice in the area. According to family records, the first member of the Yanagida family to settle in Isemachi was Teizō's ancestor Ryūboku. Born in Harima, he served as a doctor to the daimyo Asano Takuminokami (1667–1701). After the demise of Asano in 1701, Ryūboku settled in Kōzuke. The Yanagidas' large house was situated on what is now the main street of Nakanojō-machi. Through a flourishing medical practice and careful management, the family gradually became quite wealthy. Teizō was a valuable associate for the struggling Chōei.

Little is known about Teizō's education.[71] Presumably, he learned his work from his father. In addition to this, he appears to have specialized in fevers, under the tutelage of a man called Hagi Zaemon, and learned calligraphy with a man called Ryōko. Teizō's father, Yanagida Ryūan, was acquainted with Itō Chūtai, who has already been introduced as the copier of the lecture notes of 1833. Chūtai was a physician from Saku in neighboring Shinano who trained in the *koihō* school under one of its leading physicians, Yoshimasu Nangai (1750–1813). Chūtai was also interested in Western medicine and made many copies of Western medical books. He

---

70. Maruyama, *Gunma no ishi*, p. 148.

71. This account is based mostly on the information contained in the preface to Kanai, ed., *Yanagida Teizō no Tenpō kiji*.

opened a medical practice in Itahanashuku, Kōzuke, and seems to have associated closely with physicians from Nakanojō.[72] It was Itō who wrote the inscription on Yanagida Ryūan's gravestone when he died in 1824. Since Itō was also Keisaku's teacher, perhaps Teizō learned from him too.

The relationship between Teizō and Chōei is, in terms of personal correspondence, the best-documented relationship of all the three Kōzuke physicians. There are seven letters addressed to Teizō included in the *Takano Chōei den*. Perhaps more than anything, this is a reflection of the warmth of their friendship. Teizō appears to have made a habit of sending Chōei a gift of pheasants every year, as may be seen from the following letter he received in thanks: "Thank you again, for the four pheasants, this year as every year. I cooked and enjoyed them immediately. However, it is a long way, and I am always deeply grateful for your kindness."[73] Despite the risks involved in keeping documents related to Chōei following his arrest and escape from prison, a large number of Chōei's works were found hidden in Teizo's home after he died.[74]

Like Sōtei, Teizō was a welcome source of financial support for Chōei. As we have seen, in 1838, when his house burned down, Chōei called upon Teizō, just as he did Sōtei, for financial help. In a letter dated the fourth month of 1838, Chōei went into great detail about the fire and the damage to his house and asked Teizō to send wood for reconstructing it. He claimed to have heard of the existence of a lumber business quite close to Isemachi and that buying from there would be much cheaper than purchasing timber in Edo. In any case, as can be seen from the letter written to Sōtei quoted above, Chōei seems to have had no money on hand.

During the Tenpō years, Teizō kept a journal, the *Tenpō kiji*, which included many anecdotes, copies of official documents, and snippets about current affairs. The most interesting entries are those concerning the plight of the common people during the Tenpō famine, and these will be discussed further in the following chapter. Teizō was probably inspired to write these passages by his

---

72. Aoki, "Sōmō no rangaku," pp. 251–53.
73. Takano Chōun, *Takano Chōei den*, p. 326.
74. Kanai, *Takano Chōei to Agatsuma*, p. 18.

work on Chōei's *Treatise on Two Things for the Relief of Famine*. The journal is also important because it demonstrates the extent to which Teizō was able to obtain information about events in the capital and elsewhere.

Teizō often seems to have stayed the night at Keisaku's house in Yokō village. This is a useful indication of the warmth of their friendship; their houses were separated only by about twenty minutes' brisk walk. There is evidence in Keisaku's library notebook that he was lending Teizō books as early as 1827. As suggested above, the two may also have been connected by Keisaku's teacher, Itō Chūtai. One scholar has suggested that the friendship between Teizō and Keisaku may have cooled somewhat in later years, because whereas Keisaku chose to live quietly as a farmer and village official, Teizō displayed a very critical view of political affairs in his *Tenpō kiji*.[75] This idea may be thoroughly refuted, however, by a careful reading of Keisaku's diary. Not only did Keisaku attend Teizō as he lay critically ill in 1855, he continued to visit and treat his family members with similar compassion long after his friend's death (see Chapter 4).

Takahashi Keisaku was youngest of the three physicians, and the only one to live on into the Meiji period. He was born into a farming family in the village of Yokō (present-day Nakanojō) in 1799. His main farming interests were in grains, beans, and silk, although early in his life farming seems to have taken second place to medicine. It has been suggested that Keisaku's interest in studying Dutch could have sprung from an interest in silk production,[76] though this factor compares poorly with the influence of his teacher of medicine, Itō Chūtai. Keisaku's ancestors had served as village headmen; thus the Takahashi family was a well-established presence in the village.

Keisaku displayed an interest in learning from a young age and studied Chinese medicine under Itō Chūtai. Keisaku seems to have entered Chōei's school, the Daikandō in Edo, in 1831, one year after it was established. Significantly, this is also the year in which Fukuda Sōtei is believed to have first invited Chōei to Kōzuke,

---

75. Tabata, "Bakumatsu ni okeru ichi chihō ran'i no jiseki ni tsuite," p. 58.
76. Ibid., p. 45.

which suggests that Keisaku may well have followed him to Edo at this time. Within a year, he had become head student, responsible for transcribing Chōei's lessons and lecturing in his absence. The notes he took at the 1833 lectures may have been in this official capacity as Chōei's chief assistant. Accounts differ as to when he returned to Kōzuke. The inscription on his grave suggests it was 1838 and refers to some kind of internal dispute within the school that encouraged him to leave. The inscription also claims that Chōei had received an invitation to become a doctor to a particular daimyo and encouraged Keisaku to take the position in his place, but Keisaku refused and returned home. Maruyama Kiyoyasu has suggested that this inscription is somewhat unreliable and argued for a much earlier date of 1834 for Keisaku's return to the village. He based his argument on an examination of the kind of materials Keisaku had been reading.[77]

Upon his return, Keisaku continued his medical work and began to teach. He kept a record of the books that he borrowed and lent, which provides an interesting picture of the people with whom he associated. He also made some translations of Dutch books, which he used in his teaching but did not publish.[78] Keisaku kept a diary faithfully until he died, with the significant exception of the years 1840–52, 1859, and 1866. The reasons for these lapses will be discussed in detail in Chapter 4. Suffice to say here that the first one implies a deep personal reaction to Chōei's imprisonment, which discouraged him even from practicing medicine. During this period, Keisaku was involved in farming activities and village affairs, becoming village headman in 1853. He returned to medical work only after Chōei's death. In later life, Keisaku taught actively and was involved in immunizing his community against smallpox. He was also deeply involved in poetry and calligraphy circles.

There has been much speculation as to whether Chōei visited the Kōzuke physicians again after his escape from prison in 1844. Local legend and oral histories have it that Chōei hid in several places close to Nakanojō. For example, it is said that Sōtei's pupil

---

77. Maruyama, *Gunma no ishi*, p. 138.

78. For example, a book called *Garamumachika* and books by ten Haaf and Benjamin Hobson (see Chapter 4).

Gentan hid Chōei near the village of Mishima, where he lived, in a small pavilion devoted to the god Jizō. In an inn called the Nabeya, in the middle of Nakanojō, there lived a man by the name of Tamura Hachirōemon, who, because of his involvement in a local disturbance during the Tenpō years, found himself in the same prison as Chōei. His daughter Riu later testified that she could remember Chōei being hidden in the storehouse when she was a child.[79] A letter and paintings by Chōei and a measuring spoon said to have been used by him are kept in the inn today. Keisaku, too, is said to have hidden Chōei in a temple, the Bunshuin, near his home in Yokō village. Although it is impossible to determine if these accounts are fact or fiction inspired by the mystery surrounding Chōei's whereabouts, it is difficult to believe that he would not have taken the opportunity to pass through Kōzuke on the journey he made to the north after his escape. Looking at the landscape around Nakanojō too, which even now retains a certain remoteness, it is easy to imagine it was the perfect place to hide.

It is perhaps most difficult to account for Chōei's first visit to the region. As may be seen from his own life, it was common for students from rural areas to travel to Edo to study. Yet the scholar made efforts to travel to Nakanojō himself, and at least one of these journeys was something like a lecture tour. Was it simply the strength of Fukuda Sōtei's personal reputation that lured him there? Or, like so many other Edo scholars in his time, did he find the prospect of some financial patronage too good to refuse?

In answer to this, there is some evidence to suggest that Chōei already had some personal connections in Kōzuke before 1831. As we already know, Chōei's younger cousin Yōrin (Genryō) was staying in Kōzuke during the 1830s. Yōrin appears to have been based in Shibukawa, not Nakanojō, but Chōei nevertheless asked Teizō to look after him in an early letter dated 1831.[80]

Murakami Zuiken (1798–1865) is usually thought of as the pioneer of Western medicine in Kōzuke. Zuiken settled in Sakaimachi in 1828, but before this, he studied with Yoshida Chōshuku (also Chōei's teacher) in Edo, and is also said to have studied with Sie-

79. Kanai, *Takano Chōei to Agatsuma*, p. 12.
80. Takano Chōun, *Takano Chōei den*, p. 253.

bold in Nagasaki. At least one letter written by Chōei to Zuiken exists to testify to their acquaintance.[81]

More important, Chōei was acquainted with a physician by the name of Kogure Shun'an (1798–1867), from Tadanori, another village near Nakanojō. Shun'an studied under such major figures as Hirata Atsutane, Hanaoka Seishū, and Yoshida Chōshuku. Following Chōshuku's death in 1824, Shun'an also studied under Chōei, who, as we have seen, took over the teaching at the school for a short time in an emergency capacity. In Nakanojō, there is evidence in Keisaku's lending book that Shun'an borrowed a book from Keisaku in 1827; the two were obviously acquainted. It is therefore highly probable that Shun'an was a key figure in introducing Keisaku and the Kōzuke physicians to Chōei.[82] This unfortunately does not explain Chōei's connection to Fukuda Sōtei, if indeed it was Sōtei that first invited him. The question also remains as to why Sōtei was conspicuously absent from the lecture series in 1833.

On the other hand, there are other reasons why Chōei might have wished to visit the Nakanojō region, both as a physician of Western medicine and as a tourist. Were there indeed, as local historian Kanai Kōsaku has suggested, geographical and economic factors that predisposed Nakanojō to become a rural center for Western learning?[83]

The Physicians and Medicinal Plants

In his *Takano Chōei den*, Takano Chōun claimed that on one of Chōei's visits to Kōzuke, he, Sōtei, and the others went to Mt. Haruna together to collect herbs.[84] If this was the case, then Chōei had a good reason for visiting the area in person.

Fukuda Sōtei's great-grandfather was supposed to have been interested in botany, a factor that, it is said, tempted him to settle in

---

81. See ibid., p. 313.
82. Kanai, *Takano Chōei to Agatsuma*, p. 24.
83. Kanai, "Rangaku to waga Nakanojōmachi," pp. 1106–15.
84. Takano Chōun, *Takano Chōei den*, p. 310.

Sawatari and become a physician.[85] According to local documents, the reason behind the construction of Sawatari bridge in 1721 was that the famous botanist Niwa Seihaku (1700–52) was visiting on his search for medicinal herbs. Seihaku had been ordered at this time by the shogun Yoshimune to travel all over the country and collect medicinal herbs for study. One enthusiastic local scholar even went so far as to suggest that Seihaku probably stayed in the Fukuda inn when he visited.[86] The literary figure Hirasawa Kyokuzan (1733–91) also visited Sawatari, and wrote in his *Manyū bunsō* that he met travelers on the road, each carrying medicinal herbs in his hand.[87]

Chōei appears to have had a particular interest in the collection and cultivation of medicinal herbs, especially ones related to Western medicine, which he shared with the Kōzuke physicians. In 1833, while studying in Chōei's school, Keisaku compiled a book of the medicines his teacher commonly used in his treatments, which he called *Zuikōdō hōshū* (Collection of treatments at Zuikō's school).[88] Chōei himself translated two volumes on Western pharmacology, which included the Latin and sometimes Chinese names of drugs and detailed explanations of their uses.[89]

Further indication of a shared interest in medicinal herbs can be seen in a letter written by Chōei to Yanagida Teizō in the fourth month of 1838:

For several years, we have been interested in procuring the seeds to some Dutch medicinal plants, and gradually began to approach various interpreters (*tsūji*) about the matter. Through various agents they sent a request to Holland, and when the Dutch came on their official visit to Edo this year, they brought the seeds of about twenty different varieties of plants. Since it would have been a great shame if they gave them to anyone else, we bought them all up with eighteen-carat gold. According to the law, we planted them immediately. The seven varieties listed below

85. Karasawa, *Agatsuma shichō*, p. 158.
86. Kanai, "Fukuda Kōsai no rangaku no michi to Agatsuma rangaku," p. 33.
87. Ibid.
88. Zuikō was one of Chōei's pen names.
89. Both these works may be found in Takano Chōei Zenshū Kankō Kai, ed., *Takano Chōei zenshū*, vol. 1.

have already begun to sprout: *yaratsupa, soikuruorutoru, uirude salaate, shiuringu, tokerekerusu, supina, jiirootebiitooruteru.*[90]

We also planted some saffron, but it is yet to sprout. Of the plants, the *yaratsupa* is especially useful. Two stalks are sprouting. We should be able to harvest a great many seeds in the sixth and seventh months.

The "afternoon lady"[91] now has many seeds. The chrysanthemum seeds are said to be the first in Japan. Although nothing has grown apart from these, I am very hopeful.

I hope in the seventh month I will be able to give you some seeds from the *yaratsupa* as a token of my thanks for the timber. However, this is strictly confidential, so please do not speak of it to others.[92]

The "we" of this letter probably refers to members of the Shō-shikai. Watanabe Kazan, with the help of interpreters, is known to have interviewed the head of the Dutch factory, Niemann, when he made this journey to Edo in 1838;[93] so perhaps the seeds were obtained through these connections. Although these plants, apart from the *yaratsupa* (jalap), may give the impression of being ordinary vegetables rather than medicinal plants, beet and cress at least had a medicinal history in Europe, and spinach and sorrel were both used as potherbs.[94] Furthermore, the Dutch had their own vegetable garden in Dejima, which indicates that the seeds for these plants were possibly obtained within Japan. There is evidence that the Dutch were eating spinach, at least, on the island.[95]

Apart from this letter's depiction of the professional and personal nature of the relationship between Chōei and Teizō, it is an extremely important example of the direct role *ranpō* physicians such as Chōei had in introducing new plants, and the way in which

---

90. The identification of these plants has proved difficult. The following is a list of my best guesses: *yaratsupa* = jalap, *soikuruorutoru* = *suikerwortel* (sugar beet), *uirude salaate* = *wilde salade* (wild lettuce), *shiuringu* = *zuring* (sorrel), *tokerekerusu* = *ker* (cress), *supina* = *spinazie* (spinach), *jiirootebiitooruteru* = *kroot-beetwortel* (beetroot).

91. *Mirabilis japala.*

92. Takano Chōun, *Takano Chōei den*, pp. 320–23.

93. Satō, *Watanabe Kazan*, pp. 124–35.

94. Bailey, *The Standard Cyclopedia of Horticulture*; Hyams, *Plants in the Service of Man*; Simmonds, ed., *Evolution of Crop Plants*.

95. See Yanai, ed., *Nagasaki Dejima no shokubunka.*

personal networks such as that between Chōei and the Kōzuke physicians facilitated the dispersal of the plants among the medical community. It is unclear in what sense Chōei wished this information to be confidential. Since he wrote that they planted the seeds "according to the law," it would not appear that the purchase of the seeds in itself was illegal. Perhaps he simply did not wish Teizō to tell his friends of the seeds because he could not extend the same favor to them all.

In another letter addressed to his cousin Yōrin, Chōei asked him to tell Kogure (Sokuō) of Shibukawa that the arnica flowers near Mizusawa were still in full bloom and that he should make sure he collected a quantity of them immediately.

Sōtei, too, appears to have actively encouraged the cultivation of medicinal plants. In a letter he wrote to Mochizuki Shunsai, he answered his colleague's request to explain the cultivation of aloes, licorice, and other herbs. Sōtei encouraged Shunsai to plant as many as possible, ending the letter by saying: "if you intend to plant a lot, I am happy to come over and advise you."[96] The exchange of practical information such as that concerning the cultivation and collection of medicinal herbs was part of the support the physicians provided for one another.

Beyond Kōzuke

In a discussion of the reasons why Takano Chōei came to be connected to the Nakanojō region, Kanai Kōsaku suggested two important factors: the region had an abundance of medicinal herbs, and it was a popular thermal springs resort.[97] There were indeed many physicians in the area, several of whom became interested in Western learning.[98] It is interesting to note that in nineteenth-century England too, physicians tended to be concentrated in spa, cathedral, and seaside towns.[99] I have discussed earlier the social and economic

---

96. Kanai, "Takano Chōei monka Nakanojōmachi Mochizuki Shunsai no hizō monjo o haiken shite," pp. 22–23.

97. Kanai, *Takano Chōei to Agatsuma*, p. 56.

98. Kanai, "Rangaku to waga Nakanojōmachi," pp. 1107–8.

99. Waddington, "General Practitioners and Consultants in Early Nineteenth Century England," p. 173.

factors, such as the rise of commercial medicine and travel for pleasure, that contributed to the prosperity of medicine in the Nakanojō region at this time. These conditions, as well as the reputation of Fukuda Sōtei and the possibility of financial backing, would seem more than sufficient to have aroused Chōei's interest.

That Chōei did form a connection to the physicians in this rural area is a significant example of the way knowledge of Western medicine, transmitted by means of personal networks, was penetrating peripheral areas of Japan. Indeed, the Kōzuke physicians were by no means an isolated phenomenon. By the first half of the nineteenth century, *ranpō* medicine was alive and well in the countryside all over Japan. It had a place not only in the houses of great daimyo in the provinces but also in villages. A surprising number of these doctors were wealthy commoners who had trained in the great cities and returned to their local regions to practice.

For many years, the presence of Western-style *ranpō* doctors in the countryside was virtually ignored by historians. This began to change late in the 1960s with the work of Tasaki Tetsurō, who pointed to the example of rural doctors in Mikawa province (Aichi prefecture). His essays were eventually published collectively as *Zaison no rangaku* in 1985.[100] During the 1970s and 1980s, similar studies began to appear, focusing mainly on the history of smallpox inoculations and the local history of *rangaku* in terms of practical learning.[101] Recent collections of essays have tried to examine the extent to which *rangaku* had permeated the countryside, though the picture is still far from complete.[102]

According to a poll made in 1874, early in the Meiji period, there were 28,262 doctors in Japan. Of this number, 5,247, or roughly 18 percent, professed to be doctors of Western medicine. Of these *ranpō* doctors, 258 were based in Tokyo, meaning that some 4,989 others were based in outlying regions.[103] This suggests that Western

---

100. Tasaki, *Zaison no rangaku.*

101. Aoki, *Zaison rangaku no kenkyū*, pp. 3–8.

102. For example, Tasaki, ed., *Zaison rangaku no tenkai.*

103. Kōseisho Imukyoku, ed., *Isei hyakunenshi*, appendix p. 45. The figures for Tokyo are quoted in Tasaki, "Yōgaku no denpan, fukyū," pp. 57–58. Note that there is a misprint in Tasaki's figures.

medicine already had quite a firm base in regional areas even before Meiji-period legislation began to require doctors to train in Western medical techniques.

Another important clue to the extent of the *rangaku* network comes from the registers of students kept at prominent *rangaku* schools. Aoki Toshiyuki has made a study of the origins of some 5,134 medical students listed on the rolls of 12 famous *ranpō* schools.[104] According to his research, of 69 Japanese historical provinces, only one, the island of Iki, had no students in these schools. Even the island of Sado boasted 27 students of Western medicine, hardly less than Kōzuke, which had 30. By comparison, the provinces with the largest numbers of *ranpō* students were Mino and Bizen, with over 200 students each, mostly in the schools founded by Hanaoka Seishū and Ema Shunrei (1747–1838). Thus, when seen against the background of the large number of doctors studying Western medicine in other provinces, Kōzuke was far from outstanding.

Since the register for Takano Chōei's school, the Daikandō in Edo, is unfortunately not extant, Keisaku and friends are not included in this figure. Sōtei and Teizō in any case did not undertake formal study in Chōei's school and are unlikely to have been listed. So there are several difficulties in using school registers to measure the number of *ranpō* doctors, and they must be used only as a general guide. From Aoki's examination alone, it is also impossible to determine how many of the students listed on these registers returned to their homes to practice medicine in the countryside. There is reason to suspect that many of them did.

Tasaki Tetsurō's research, which focused mainly on *ranpō* doctors in the province of Mikawa, has suggested that there was a trend among doctors of farmer origin to commence their studies with Chinese medicine and branch out into Western medicine later in their careers.[105] Most rural doctors went away from their homes to study in private medical schools for a period of ten years or so, after which they returned to succeed their fathers in medical prac-

---

104. Aoki, *Zaison rangaku no kenkyū*, pp. 16–17. Aoki includes Hanaoka Seishū's school, although he was not strictly a *ranpō* physician.

105. Tasaki, *Chihō chishikijin no keisei*, p. 278.

tice at the local level. Although not all of them studied in Edo, the physicians in Kōzuke appear to fit this general pattern.

Tasaki argued that the tendency for these doctors to return home was due to a strong sense of local loyalty and the absence of a developed meritocracy that would allow them to aspire to distinguished careers in the cities. He also suggested that such doctors had a strong sense of responsibility and self-awareness of their role as village leaders.[106]

Sometimes, village officials may have sent their sons to study medicine for political reasons. Aoki gave the example of a doctor in Matsushiro domain, in Shinshū, who was born into a wealthy farming family whose members often had to vie for appointment as village headman. As the eldest son, Miyahara Ryōseki was sent to study medicine in Nagasaki for three years. Although he returned to the village, Ryōseki's younger brother later took over as village headman, leaving Ryōseki free to practice medicine. During the Tenpō famine, Ryōseki was congratulated by his domain for boiling and serving two days' worth of rice porridge to more than 600 starving villagers. Aoki has suggested that having a doctor in the family helped village leaders to solve problems of health and poverty in the village and hence maintain their popularity. Eventually, Ryōseki was given an official position as doctor to the Matsushiro domain.[107]

By returning to their villages, doctors did not cut themselves off from the outside world or even from the possibility of promotion. Some domains went so far as to begin to promote the training of village doctors. Ryōseki's domain of Matsushiro was one of the few domains to implement a form of medical licensing. It did this by offering official lectures once a month and encouraging those from outlying areas to attend. The lectures were based on Chinese learning, for this was seen to be a necessary base for both Chinese and Western medicine. Farmers from all levels applied to attend, although those from powerful families had certain advantages.[108]

---

106. Ibid., p. 285.
107. Aoki, *Zaison rangaku no kenkyū*, pp. 244–54.
108. Ibid., pp. 257–74.

Lessons in medicine could also be taken via correspondence. This is well demonstrated by the letters between Chōei and Sōtei, discussed above. For people separated by distance, letters were a means of maintaining and reinforcing social relationships. For many country students who studied in the cities, they were a lifeline that kept them in touch with their teachers and colleagues after they returned to the countryside. Chōei's adoptive father, Gensai, is an interesting early example of this, for he continued to exchange letters with his famous teacher Sugita Genpaku and colleague Ōtsuki Gentaku long after he returned to his native Mizusawa.[109]

Miyaji has noted the example of Tsuboi Shinryō (1823–1904), who, from his origins as the second son of a doctor in Takaoka in the province of Etchū, became the adopted son of Tsuboi Shindō and had a prestigious career as a Bakufu doctor, serving the shogun Yoshinobu. From 1846 until 1877, Shinryō sent detailed letters to his elder brother, who, after his studies, had returned home to succeed to the practice in Takaoka. The letters were full of all the Edo news and current affairs; their nature changed only after 1874, when Shinryō began to send a newspaper instead. Shinryō also sent books and information on publications, and even other documents so that his brother might understand the books.[110] This is a powerful example of the role of letters as a source of information in early modern Japan.

In the context of European history, Pearl has written a short article about the importance of correspondence in the spread of scientific information in early modern France. Pearl argued that, unlike books, letters were not subject to censorship, and they did not take a long time to publish, meaning that they could be filled with the latest information. Furthermore, the author argued, "newly received letters were read aloud at gatherings of interested scholars, and copies were made and forwarded to others."[111] One innovative provincial scholar, Nicolas Fabri de Peiresc (1580–1637),

---

109. According to Satō Shōsuke, however, none of the extant letters concern medical matters. See Satō, *Takano Chōei*, p. 10.

110. Miyachi, *Bakumatsu ishinki no bunka to jōhō*, pp. 177–212.

111. Pearl, "The Role of Personal Correspondence," p. 107.

was able to organize an observation of the same lunar eclipse in 1635 in Paris, Aix, Rome, Naples, Cairo, Aleppo, and Quebec, all by letter.[112] Issues such as censorship and the length of time taken to publish were significant in Japan too, especially in the oppressive climate of the Tenpō period. Although there is no record of Chōei's letters having been read aloud, there is little doubt that their contents at least were shared among his friends in Kōzuke.

Having seen the geographical and historical setting for the relationship between Chōei and the Kōzuke physicians, let us now turn to the product of their efforts. The next chapter will examine their collaborative works and the way in which they attempted to use Western knowledge for their practical pursuits.

---

112. Ibid., p. 111.

CHAPTER 3

Famine, Epidemics, and the Social Role of Physicians

In the autumn and winter of 1836, at the height of the Tenpō famine, Chōei busied himself writing two works on ways to relieve the plight of the common people. Perhaps best described as pamphlets, they were inspired by conversations held with the physicians in Kōzuke. Indeed, it was shortly after Chōei visited the group in the eighth month of that year that he began to write them. The physicians' joint efforts resulted in the publication of two pamphlets: *Treatise on Two Things for the Relief of Famine* and *Methods of Avoiding Epidemic Diseases.*[1] In the first of these, Chōei described a special type of buckwheat and the white potato and their possible role in warding off starvation when other crops failed. In the latter, he gave practical information aimed at preventing the diseases that tended to strike after famine.

These documents serve as examples of the way knowledge from Western sources spread through social networks and was interpreted, adapted, and used for practical purposes at the local level.

---

1. *Treatise on Two Things for the Relief of Famine* (*Kyūkō nibutsukō*) in Takano Chōei Zenshū Kankō Kai, ed., *Takano Chōei zenshū*, 4: 1–33; *Methods of Avoiding Epidemic Diseases* (*Hieki yōhō*) in ibid., 1: 217–31. *Treatise on Two Things for the Relief of Famine* was reprinted by the Gunma prefectural government in 1883, and it is this version (in handwritten text) that is reproduced in the *Zenshū*.

This chapter explores through these writings what Chōei did with Western knowledge on his own terms and in his own time and place. It unfolds the influence of practical learning (*jitsugaku*) on the way *rangaku* scholarship was applied to problems of famine and disease, not only in this case but in others.

Furthermore, *Treatise on Two Things for the Relief of Famine* and *Methods of Avoiding Epidemic Diseases* help to form a picture of the kinds of problems the famine created for common people and the physicians who tried to treat them. They supply clues as to how physicians perceived their social role as intellectuals and as protectors of community health, both as authors and transmitters of medical information. The two documents are translated in full in the Appendixes. In order best to understand the context of these works—that is, the reasons Chōei and the physicians utilized the new knowledge in the way they did—it is important to look first at the historical background to this period of famine.[2]

The Tenpō Famine

The Tenpō famine, the last of three so-called great famines in Japan's early modern period, lasted seven years, from Tenpō 3 (1832) until the autumn of Tenpō 10 (1838).[3] It was caused by a series of crop failures due to unseasonably damp and cold weather. To be successful in growing rice, which was an important food as well as the basis of the taxation system, two conditions need to be satisfied: one, that there is enough water; and two, that the temperature is warm (usually no less than twenty degrees centigrade in summer).[4] In the Kantō and Tōhoku areas, where summer temperatures were often cooler than was required for rice growing, crop failure was a common occurrence. This problem was usually known as *reigai*, or "cold damage." In contrast, drought was more often the source of

---

2. Unfortunately, it has proved impossible to trace the Western works on which the Japanese doctors based their information. Chōei himself gives no clues, and the works are not included in bibliographies of Dutch works translated in Japan.

3. Kikuchi, *Kinsei no kikin*, pp. 1–5.

4. Arakawa, *Saigai no rekishi*, p. 67.

crop failure in the west of Japan.[5] There were considerable regional differences in harvests even during famine years. In 1836, which was the most devastating year of the Tenpō famine, not only areas in the north, but even Shikoku and the areas around the Inland Sea were affected. As a whole, the country averaged around 2 percent of a regular harvest.[6]

That the people were starving could not, however, be blamed entirely on the inclement weather. The complex economic relationship between the domains and the central government, the volatility of the price of rice, and the failure to store enough of it were some of the factors in this complex and tragic situation. It has been argued, for example, that starvation was first and foremost a problem for those people who were not necessarily poor but were not self-sufficient and could not afford to buy food at exorbitant prices.[7] As will be seen later, Chōei, too, commented that for some, a day's wage was not enough to buy a day's food supply.[8] Sometimes economists have referred to this ability of a person to buy sufficient food at the current price as the "entitlement" to food.[9] The use of this concept serves as a reminder of the need to consider, when examining famine, not only crop failure but the rice market and the various ways in which it was manipulated.

Indeed, some people were able to benefit from fluctuations in the price of rice. We can see this in the diary of Kawai Koume, the wife of a Confucian scholar living in Wakayama. Although she noted the high rice prices in her diary in 1837, she did not appear to be suffering any discomfort. On the contrary, it appears her family was able to profit from the high prices at which her husband's rice stipend was sold.[10] As will be seen later, it is clear that Chōei and his associates, too, were far from going hungry. At the other end of the social scale, in addition to the regular forms of discrimination

---

5. Kikuchi, *Kinsei no kikin*, pp. 12–14.

6. Uesugi, "Tenpō no kikin to bakuhan taisei no hōkai," p. 106.

7. Amino, *Zoku Nihon no rekishi o yominaosu*, pp. 176–81.

8. See Appendix A, p. 184.

9. Walter and Schofield, eds., *Famine, Disease and the Social Order in Early Modern Society*, p. 14.

10. Hanley, *Everyday Things in Premodern Japan*, p. 89.

that they suffered, *eta* (untouchables) were sometimes denied the aid that was distributed to other poor people in times of famine.[11]

Nor was the famine simply a problem of the rice harvest. The extent to which ordinary farmers ate rice is hotly debated. It appears to have become increasingly common as a staple food over time, especially in the cities. In the countryside, people probably ate a mixture of barley, millet, and some rice to glue it all together.[12] As will be seen below, in areas such as Nakanojō, in Kōzuke, which was not climatically suited to growing rice, Yanagida Teizō appears to have been just as troubled by the poor quality of the barley crop as that of rice. He did at the same time take a careful interest in the fluctuations of the rice market. He and Takahashi Keisaku alike made detailed observations of the market price of rice in their journals.

Hunger was not the only suffering inflicted by the famine. It was commonly understood in the Edo period that famines were often followed by outbreaks of epidemic disease. In his writings, Chōei suggested that the strange eating habits people adopted in times of famine may have been a source of intestinal upset and disease. He went on to note that epidemics were far more damaging to people than famine.[13]

Modern historical interpretations of the situation are less clear. As Jannetta explains, it is often difficult to distinguish between famines and epidemics using historical records, because "1) people who suffer from severe malnutrition may actually die of infection, or they may exhibit symptoms similar to those caused by certain acute infectious diseases; and 2) the mortality rate from some infectious diseases may be higher among people who are malnourished."[14]

In Tokugawa Japan, the impact of epidemics has been interpreted by some scholars from population records, in which the number of deaths was highest in the year after severe crop failure.[15]

---

11. Matsuoka, "Kikin to sabetsu," p. 132.

12. Hanley, "Tokugawa Society: Material Culture, Standard of Living, and Life-Styles," p. 683.

13. See Appendixes, pp. 184, 206.

14. Jannetta, *Epidemics and Mortality in Early Modern Japan*, p. 173.

15. Kikuchi, *Kinsei no kikin*, pp. 12–14.

Perhaps this was because people's immune systems were weakened by malnutrition, making them more susceptible to disease. Yet, as Walter and Schofield have argued, nutritional status is complex. It is not simply related to the quantity of food available, but also to work and living conditions, as well as the level of exposure to disease and parasites. The immune system fails only in conditions of extreme malnutrition, and in the case of some diseases, moderate malnutrition may even help. Only in extreme circumstances—for example, if people began turning to poisonous or polluted foods—did they run the risk of a fatal digestive infection. Therefore, the link that Chōei described between famine and epidemic disease may have been more significantly influenced by a greater exposure to disease caused by chaotic social circumstances and migratory behavior than by unusual eating habits.[16]

It has also been suggested that the mortality crisis in 1830s Japan may have been a subsistence crisis rather than the result of epidemic disease. Records found of an epidemic in the village of Hida during the Tenpō famine described an acute diarrhea, which may also be a symptom displayed by the human body in the final stages of starvation.[17] This evidence, however, is not reinforced by that of Chōei, who, while stressing the importance of a clean digestive system, made no mention of diarrhea.

Chōei's treatments for epidemic fevers included those for symptoms such as headache, insomnia, pain from intestinal worms, and a constricted chest. He advised readers to diagnose epidemic fever when "there is an epidemic fever in the vicinity and the patient complains of heavy limbs, headache, feels a terrible chill, and breaks out in a sweat."[18] As has been observed for the situation in southeastern England, the premodern conception of "epidemic fever" was very general and may have included any number of diseases that induced a feverish state, including enteric fevers and

---

16. Walter and Schofield, eds., *Famine, Disease and the Social Order in Early Modern Society*, pp. 18–20, 55–57.

17. Jannetta, "Famine Mortality in Nineteenth-Century Japan: The Evidence from a Temple Death Register."

18. See Appendix B, p. 209.

influenza.[19] If Chōei's patients were suffering from acute malnutrition as well as from infectious diseases, the strong purges that he recommended were probably the last thing that their exhausted bodies needed.[20]

Chōei clearly seems to have thought that his patients were suffering from an epidemic disease, writing that "in this period of peace and prosperity, the administrators have a policy of charitable alms, and the people are thereby saved from starvation."[21] Although this assertion may have been simply designed to curry favor with government officials, a further investigation of the link between famine and disease in early modern Japan is clearly required.

Assessing the impact of the Tenpō famine and the disease by which it was accompanied can be seen as forming part of an ongoing debate about the general level of well-being in premodern Japan. In the words of Conrad Totman, scholars can be divided into "those who see Tokugawa rural history as essentially an optimistic story of progress and human betterment" and those who "view it as a grim account of human degradation and immiseration that generated revolutionary rage."[22] In many cases, such debates are also connected with population studies. Most historical demographers believe that during the Tokugawa period there was a large burst of population growth during the first half of the period, particularly during the seventeenth century, after which it slowed, or continued to grow only very slowly, until after the beginning of the Meiji period.[23] The reasons given for the slowing population growth, however, are highly contested.[24] In accounts by scholars belonging to Totman's latter classification, famine and epidemics have been commonly cited as significant factors influencing the "stagnant" population during this period. Such historians often focus on the most seriously affected areas in the north of Japan to

---

19. Dobson, *Contours of Death and Disease in Early Modern England*, p. 459.

20. See Kiple, ed., *The Cambridge World History of Human Disease*; Davey, Halliday, and Hirst, eds., *Human Biology and Health*.

21. Appendix B, p. 199.

22. Totman, "Tokugawa Peasants: Win, Lose, or Draw," p. 463.

23. Totman, *Early Modern Japan*, p. 250.

24. Ibid., p. 250.

demonstrate the devastating effect of famine.[25] Practices such as infanticide and cannibalism are cited to show the terrible lengths to which people went in order to survive. In the other school of thought, scholars such as Hanley and Yamamura have argued that overall population figures do not reflect the fact that there were regional differences in population growth. When these are taken into account, it appears that the population was not stagnant, but continued to grow (albeit slowly) throughout the eighteenth and nineteenth centuries. While Hanley and Yamamura acknowledge that famines had a negative impact on population, particularly in the Tōhoku region, their studies found that famine and disease were not sufficient to explain the low rate of population growth. They suggested that people controlled reproduction intentionally, with the aim of increasing their standard of living, and were hesitant to attribute the low rate of increase to the ravages of famine.[26] More recently, Totman has argued that population issues need to be addressed in view of ecological history. He suggested that the Edo period population had reached levels at the limits of what the ecosystem could support, and the slowing population growth and frugal existence lived by so many people were reflections of the need to make do with the resources they had.[27]

Images of Famine in Yanagida Teizō's *Tenpō kiji*

Whatever the impact in concrete terms, the extent to which the Tenpō famine was written about in the literature of the time gives an indication of its social impact. Even if these stories were exaggerated or based on hearsay, the very fact that they were written is important. Yanagida Teizō of Isemachi was one of the many who felt compelled to write about the suffering he witnessed around him, as people struggled to find enough to eat. His journal, which

---

25. For example, Nakajima, *Kikin Nihonshi*, pp. 118–21.

26. Hanley and Yamamura, *Economic and Demographic Change in Preindustrial Japan, 1600–1868.*

27. Totman, "Tokugawa Peasants," p. 470.

he called *Tenpō kiji* (Tenpō annals),[28] contained many anecdotes about the famine. His sympathetic descriptions touched on different aspects, sometimes sad, sometimes amusing, sometimes astonishing. The stories are too numerous to quote at length, but some representative ones are included here. The first example is a local story from Yamada village. It is followed by one concerning the prostitutes in the famous Yoshiwara quarter in Edo.

In the autumn of 1836, there had been a series of thefts of millet at night, so watchmen were placed in huts to guard the crop. In Yamada village, there was an elderly couple found taking the millet in broad daylight. The owner of the field, extremely indignant, scolded them. The couple said that they had no choice but to steal because they had nothing to put in their pot to cook. It would make no difference to them whether they were given the millet or killed on the spot, they would be grateful in any case. The owner, lost for words, let them be and returned to the hut.[29]

In Edo, Yoshiwara is to be particularly pitied. When a famous establishment went to ruin, all the others in Yoshiwara were ordered by the Bakufu to give their assistance. Because the prostitutes are made to eat a rice gruel like water, they are long and thin like sick eels, scarcely able to climb the stairs. Relying on their artistic skills, getting a meal out of their guest is their main aim.[30]

On a lighter note, Teizō recounted the following:

There was a man called Matsugorō from Arikawa village whom I employed as a servant. When I took him with me on an errand, he found some excrement on the side of the road which had millet and azuki beans mixed in with it. He was extremely surprised, and exclaimed that in a year as bad as this one, the person who had left behind excrement of this nature must have been of considerable standing. "This must be indeed what it means 'to know the shape of something by its shadow'!" I laughed.[31]

Sometimes, Teizō's interests as a doctor came to the fore. For example, he made a note of successful methods of curing constipa-

---

28. The journal has been edited and published by Kanai Kōsaku. All translations are based on this version. See Kanai, ed., *Yanagida Teizō no Tenpō kiji*.
29. Ibid., p. 11.
30. Ibid., p. 20.
31. Ibid., p. 12.

tion for his future use. Teizō also demonstrated a keen interest in the kind of foods that people were eating. He recorded that arrow-root made a good substitute for wheat flour and that straw could be used to make a drink. Also noted was the fact that people in the northern province of Dewa ate dirt, by washing it and making it into something similar to a glutinous rice cake, but since Teizō made no comment, it is impossible to know what he thought of this practice. Certainly, he was suspicious of some eating habits. He warned of the danger of eating yam and sorrel[32] at the same time and also made the following observation:

People who are starving should not eat a lot of food. Also, they should not eat things made from azuki beans. There are some who have died immediately. In the eleventh month just passed someone came to Naka-nojō from Gotanda village. After he ate four or five bowls of *sekihan*,[33] he died on the outskirts of Nakanojō village.[34]

Against such a background of hunger and disease, the Tenpō years saw frequent outbreaks of civil unrest in both rural and ur-ban areas. Such forms of protest were common during times of famine. Traditionally, peasants were permitted to instigate law suits about economic matters and against corrupt local officials, as a means of defusing tension. Over the course of the Edo period, as protests became larger and more frequent in response to social changes, increasingly it was the Bakufu that took control of peas-ant protests rather than individual domain lords.[35] This was par-ticularly the case when protests crossed domain borders. This was accompanied, too, by a gradual shift in peasant consciousness in which peasants saw themselves increasingly not as subjects of their domainal lords but of the Bakufu.[36] This is why rebellions such as that of Ōshio Heihachirō, a man of samurai rank who aimed his attack directly against the Bakufu in Osaka in 1837, "shocked the

---

32. *Rumex acetosa.*

33. A dish made from glutinous rice and azuki beans, usually eaten at times of celebration.

34. Kanai, *Yanagida Teizō no Tenpō kiji*, p. 21.

35. White, "State Growth and Popular Protest in Tokugawa Japan," p. 18.

36. Ibid., p. 24.

state to its roots."[37] It provided an important impetus for the Tenpō Reforms, administrative reforms that were initiated by Mizuno Tadakuni in 1841.

Ōshio Heihachirō's famous rebellion inspired similar uprisings, including one led by Ikuta Yorozu, who, incidentally, came from Kōzuke.[38] Teizō gave detailed accounts of these rebellions in his *Tenpō kiji*. He included a complete transcription of Ōshio's call to arms, even going so far as to describe the size and cover of the book from which it was copied. Perhaps it can be said that the care with which Teizō recorded these events was a political statement in itself. It is not possible, however, to determine any particular political affiliation in his commentary. While admitting the faults of the authorities, many of whom were dismissed after Ōshio's rebellion, Teizō also noted the bravery of many on the side of the administration.

It has been suggested that rural elites in the late Edo period were displaying an increasing intellectual interest in political issues.[39] Teizō's journal appears to corroborate this idea. From his journal entries, it is obvious that he had a wide-ranging interest in current affairs and that he was well informed about events in places as far away as Edo and Osaka. This is also a reflection of the effectiveness of the transportation and communication networks discussed in the last chapter.

An interest in national political affairs did not prevent Teizō from thinking about agricultural issues closer to home. The following excerpt reflects a concern for the quality of crops as a factor in famine, an idea that is also visible through his work with Chōei on *Treatise on Two Things for the Relief of Famine*.

In 1836 it was said that barley was a huge success, the kind of harvest that happens only once in every fifty years. However, perhaps because it was an unlucky year, the barley appeared to have little moisture, and even though one ate more than usual, it was not satisfying. Everyone says that they eat more in a bad year. In 1837, too, there was as much barley as

---

37. Ibid., p. 23.
38. Totman, *Early Modern Japan*, pp. 514–18.
39. Koschmann, *The Mito Ideology*, p. 136.

usual. It would seem to be because in a bad year even though crops look good on the outside, in reality they are poor on the inside.[40]

One final passage from Teizō's diary is worth noting in relation to the topic of famine. The following quotation describes a visit made to Chōei's house in Edo. It is important because it displays the relative wealth of these men compared to those to whom they addressed their writings, and because it gives an indication of the genuine feeling Teizō seems to have had for those less fortunate, which would not allow him to make light of their predicament:

When we visited Takano Chōei's house in Kōjimachi (Edo), there was a man from Ōshū who joined in the party. This man said he knew of a way to avoid starvation in a famine year and, fanning himself, went on to say quietly that if one always ate polished rice with no dregs, cooked to perfection fish that were not oily, and ate strictly three meals a day, along with a fine *sake* according to one's taste, no matter how bad a famine year, one would never starve, at which everyone laughed heartily. However, there is a time and a place for jokes. At Takano-kata's[41] we were treated to some *sake*, which tasted so unusually good that I enquired about it. This *sake* cost fourteen *monme* of silver for one *shō*. I had drunk *sake* here and there before, but it had a strong smell and was not good *sake*. Sometimes one can find cloudy *sake*.[42]

Here it is obvious that Teizō was uncomfortable making jokes about starvation when so many people were indeed going hungry. The source of his indignation seems to have been Chōei's guest rather than Chōei himself; so we can only guess as to what the *rangaku* scholar's part in it was and whether the expensive wine belonged to him. The passage may or may not contain insight into the relationship between Teizō and Chōei; perhaps it is better interpreted as an indication of the seriousness with which Teizō regarded the famine, both in his public role as a physician and in his private life.

---

40. Kanai, *Yanagida Teizō no Tenpō kiji*, p. 17.
41. A term of respect.
42. Kanai, *Yanagida Teizō no Tenpō kiji*, p. 13.

Takano Chōei and Writings on Famine

In Edo, Chōei was also actively involved in issues to do with the famine. As described in Chapter 1, he became involved, through the influence of his employer and mentor, Watanabe Kazan, in a study group of scholars, intellectuals, and concerned officials called the Shōshikai. The group was formed by a man called Endō Katsusuke in order to discuss famine relief,[43] and many of the members were involved in Western learning.

In writing and engaging with ideas about famine, these men were adding their voices to a growing field of scholarship. The genre of *kyūkōsho* (famine books), which were books that recorded famine conditions and imparted knowledge about how to prepare for famine and what to eat to avoid starvation, developed in Japan over the eighteenth and nineteenth centuries. Produced partly as a reaction to the visible suffering caused by famine, the books were also influenced by developments in *honzōgaku*, or botanical studies.

Honzōgaku was generally considered to be an area of medicine whose purpose was to establish the correct names of plants, determine whether they had beneficial or poisonous qualities, and observe their other uses.[44] Since the *honzōgaku* tradition was imported from China, from the outset Japanese *honzōgaku* scholars spent a significant proportion of their time working out whether the plants mentioned in Chinese books existed in Japan, and if they did, equating them with their Japanese counterparts.[45] During the Tokugawa period, as it began to move from purely botanical studies to the study of natural history, *honzōgaku* began to include not only the study of medicinal herbs but also of animals, other plants, and minerals. Most books in the field continued to be based on Chinese models until Kaibara Ekiken (1630–1714) published his influential *Yamato honzō* in 1709. Following this, Western botanical books also began to attract some attention. The shogun Yoshimune, along with his promotion of other practical areas of West-

---

43. Satō, *Yōgakushi kenkyū josetsu*, pp. 134–35.
44. Fujikawa, *Nihon igakushi kōyō*, 1: 149–51.
45. Yamada, ed., *Mono no imeeji honzō to hakubutsugaku e no shōtai*, p. 34.

ern learning, displayed an interest in botanical books such as Do-donaeus's *Cruydt-Boeck* (*Herbal*). This book was deeply influential in Japan, and for the next one hundred years, many scholars attempted to read or translate it. It was not until Siebold came in 1823, bringing with him modern Western botanical books, that his students realized that Dodonaeus's famous book belonged to the past, and they focused their attention on other works.[46]

Honzōgaku had always been concerned with the identification of wild plants and determining whether they were edible. As we have seen, there was a strong interest in *honzōgaku* during the Tokugawa period, especially during the eighteenth century, and many Chinese books were brought to Japan at this time and published in Japanese versions. Some of the books were already devoted purely to the botany of foodstuffs. The purpose of these books, however, was not to assist starving people, but simply to determine the medical uses of the plants, for food was seen to be a type of medicine. From the mid-eighteenth century, developments in *honzōgaku*, agricultural writings, and natural history coincided with increasingly frequent famines in Japan, resulting in the realization that descriptions of edible plants could be used as a form of direct action to assist starving people. So famine books were born, using *honzōgaku* works for reference, but written in simpler language and focusing on practical issues such as how to prepare the plants for consumption. Since plants were usually studied only if they were useful, famine botany provided the opportunity for the examination of plants that until then had been ignored, as well as for local, experiential knowledge to become public.[47]

The first Japanese scholar to write a book directed at suffering commoners about the types of wild plants that could be gathered

---

46. For example, Takano Chōei's contemporary, Itō Keisuke, based his 1829 *Taisei honzō meiso* (The nomenclature of the Western herbals) on Thunberg's *Flora japonica*, and used the Linnaean classification system rather than that of Dodonaeus. See Vande Walle and Kasaya, eds., *Dodonaeus in Japan*, especially pp. 202–4, 270.

47. This section is based closely on Shirasugi Etsuo, "Nihon ni okeru kyūkō-sho no seiritsu to sono engen."

and eaten as a defense against famine was the physician Takebe Seian (1712–82). Although trained in Western medicine in the Katsuragawa school, Seian relied heavily on Chinese Ming-period botanical works on famine for this research. His two studies, *Minkan bikōroku* (1756) and *Bikōsōmokuzu*, published posthumously in 1833 by his son Sugita Hakugen, were frequently quoted and had a great influence on other writers in the field. The books were particularly significant because up until then, most writings on famine were concerned with good governance, and so were intended to be read by members of the ruling class rather than by the common people in order to help themselves.[48]

Takebe Seian tends to be remembered more for his close relationship with that famous founding member of *rangaku* Sugita Genpaku than for his work on famine. A set of correspondence between the two doctors in which Seian questioned Genpaku about various aspects of Western medicine was published as early as 1759. Eventually Seian sent his younger son Tsutomu to Genpaku to study with him, and in time Genpaku adopted him and gave him the name Sugita Hakugen: the same Sugita Hakugen with whom Chōei had a brief spell of study as a young student.[49]

Shirasugi counts over 80 books dealing with famine published between 1615 and 1866.[50] Included in his list were Takano Chōei's *Treatise on Two Things for the Relief of Famine* and a work called *Kyūkō benran* by Shōshikai founder Endō Katsusuke. *Rangaku* scholars, too, were beginning to use the fruits of their Western botanical scholarship to assist with the problem of famine. Even Genpaku had portrayed images of famine in his *Nochimigusa*.[51] Thus, there were many possible sources of inspiration, both within Chōei's circle of acquaintance and in the general scholarly arena, for him to write the first of his 1836 pamphlets, *Treatise on Two Things for the Relief of Famine*. The more immediate inspiration for the work, as he wrote plainly in the preface, came from his friends

---

48. Ibid., especially pp. 149–53.
49. Ibid., p. 147.
50. Ibid., pp. 167–73.
51. Kikuchi, *Kinsei no kikin*, pp. 152, 156–67.

Fukuda Sōtei and Yanagida Teizō in Kōzuke. The discussion below traces the steps by which they came to apply their knowledge of Western crops to local problems of famine.

The Treatise

Potatoes

Treatise on Two Things for the Relief of Famine was written by Chōei in Edo in 1836, shortly after a visit to Kōzuke. The preface contains a rather touching account of how it came to be written, which shows something not only of the companionable relationship between Chōei and his Kōzuke friends but of the way they tested out and exchanged ideas with each other:

In the middle of the eighth month of this year, I [Chōei] met Fukuda Sōtei of Sawatari in Jōmō. The Sōtei family has for generations been surgeons by profession, and they are very skilled in their art. Also, Sōtei reads Dutch books in order to study the subject further. I have enjoyed a warm relationship with him from the beginning, and one evening, just when our conversation was getting into full swing, he pulled out a scoop of buckwheat and showed it to me, saying,

"In general, the reason why people die in a bad year is because they do not have enough to eat. And the reason why there is not enough food is because there are not any crops that can be harvested several times a year. This buckwheat should mature three times a year. Do you not think that it would be a great treasure for the poor people?"

I was very surprised and grateful, and . . . took [the buckwheat] gladly. Later I was given a type of potato by a man called Yanagida Teizō from Isemachi in the same province.[52]

Since the Tenpō famine was due largely to the problem known as "cold damage," when summer temperatures were too cool for growing grains, Chōei saw possibilities in substituting crops that could better tolerate such weather conditions:

Consider this. Although the countries near the North Pole are intensely, bitingly cold, and there are only one or two months a year in which the

---

52. Appendix A, pp. 184–85.

ice melts, why do the people there not starve? It is because they plant things to eat that do not fear wind, cold, heat or damp. . . . When people in the countries near the North Pole choose their crops, they choose ones that grow quickly. If these crops were grown in a warm area, they would mature several times a year.[53]

Chōei went on to write in detail about the buckwheat and potato given to him by his friends, supplying details in the text about how to grow them, cook them, store them, make flour, and use them for brewing.

In writing about the usefulness of potatoes, Chōei had an important predecessor in Aoki Kon'yō (1698–1769), a famous *rangaku* forefather who had actively promoted the cultivation of sweet potatoes (*satsumaimo*) as a measure against famine. It came to the attention of the Bakufu during the Kyōhō famine (1732–33) that the low number of deaths from starvation in Satsuma domain seemed to be related to the cultivation and consumption of sweet potatoes. Kon'yō wrote a piece called *Banshokō* (Thoughts on sweet potatoes), which he submitted to a government official by the name of Ōoka in 1733 or 1734. It was intended to back up an application for public office made for him on his behalf by a friendly patron. Subsequently, he was employed by the government of shogun Yoshimune to oversee the cultivation of experimental sweet potato plots.[54]

The Kyōhō famine was caused by a combination of cold summer rain and problems with "leaf hopper" insects,[55] so the circumstances in Satsuma were slightly different from those in the north during the Tenpō famine. Nevertheless, Chōei saw advantages in the white potato over the sweet potato, claiming that it was less sensitive to cold and that it would not over-sweeten and acidify like the sweet potato. He added that "because (potatoes) have the advantage of greatly nourishing the stomach for a long time and allowing people to forget hunger, people in the West reserve their praise not for the sweet potato but only for the potato."[56]

---

53. Appendix A, pp. 184–85.
54. Sippel, "Aoki Konyō," pp. 133–34.
55. Totman, *Early Modern Japan*, pp. 236–37.
56. Appendix A, p. 197.

In much the same way as Aoki Kon'yō, Chōei seems to have been promoting the cultivation of crops that had actually been known for some time in Japan. Both sweet and white potatoes appear to have been introduced to Japan by the early seventeenth century.[57] Chōei's stance would suggest that the white potato was not very widely cultivated for human consumption. There were at least two reasons for this. Chōei's detailed instructions imply that ordinary farmers did not know how to grow potatoes, a problem Chōei seems to be addressing. There was also another factor at work here; the people were afflicted by superstitious fears:

It is commonly said that because the potato is inimical to ink, those in the literary profession should not eat it, but this is wrong. A long time ago when pumpkins and *satsumaimo* were first grown, people thought that they were incompatible with fish or meat or that they would prevent people from writing with ink, and people everywhere were afraid and did not eat them very much. Now, people eat a great deal of them, even with fish and meat, and only then do they learn of the untruth of such sayings. Potatoes are another case of this. Previously, in the West, there was a time in Bolgonie [Boulogne] (a place in France), when it was said that potatoes caused scabies, and growing them was banned. However, since then people have eaten a great deal of them and there has been no record of any ill effects, which is proof of this. Ah, although all countries differ in their climate and customs, perhaps it is not only human sentiment that is the same![58]

Thus, in some ways, Chōei's message seems to have been as much about having the courage to try new things as about the usefulness of the crops themselves. The meaning of the final sentence is not easy to determine, but it is possible to interpret it as a remarkable profession of human universalism. It is especially remarkable for a man whom at least one scholar has categorized (with little justification) as a "xenophobe."[59] Here was a man who had never left his own country, who had met only a few Europeans, and whose picture of Europe was still flawed by insufficient

---

57. Hanley, "Tokugawa Society," p. 682.
58. Appendix A, p. 197.
59. Wakabayashi, *Anti-Foreignism*, p. 61.

and misinterpreted information. Yet he seemed to be trying to say that humans have much in common and there is much that they can learn from others. Far from being overly suspicious of Europeans and their practices, it is possible to argue, on the contrary, that precisely because his information was so limited, Chōei was prone to exaggerate the benefits of Western technology and customs.

It is fascinating to see Chōei successfully explaining France's initial resistance to the consumption of potatoes. A modern scholar, Bourke, claims that the disease feared by the French was leprosy, whereas Chōei referred to scabies.[60] This was, however, presumably a problem of translation, and he has understood the gist of the problem quite well.

It is worth quoting Chōei's introduction to the potato at some length, for it demonstrates the way in which he endeavored to piece together information from various sources and interpret it in such a way as to make it easy for his readers to understand.

The origin of this tuber is also unclear. It is said that it was imported to Kai and Shinano and grown from early times. When one considers that it is called *jagataraimo* or *appura* (which is a dialect of the hinterland and probably a corruption of *aardappel*), it would seem that it was brought by the Dutch. According to Dutch books, this potato grew originally in the West Indies, after which it was grown by the French and the English. After this it was introduced to the Dutch region. Also it is very common in America, where it seems the people who have emigrated there from Europe make this tuber the staple of their diet. That is, originally, this tuber came from the West Indies and America. It was grown for the first time in Holland about 1,600 years after the beginning of the era (this is about two hundred years before the present year of 1836), and people still use it as their staple. Linnaeus (mentioned above), in his book writes about the three virtues of the potato. One, that it will flourish in areas with sandy and stony soil where other grains will not grow. Two. it will not be damaged by strong winds, heavy rains, or long frosts. Third, it is easy to grow and does not require a lot of labor. Also, an inch of land will give the yield of a foot of land, so it is also

---

60. Bourke, *"The Visitation of God"? The Potato and the Great Irish Famine*, p. 14.

called a *hasshōimo*.[61] It certainly may be said to be a good crop for a bad year.[62]

It is easy for modern historians to forget that in Europe, too, the potato was promoted originally as a supplementary food to provide against famine. It was noted particularly for its hardiness under wet and dreary conditions, that is, for precisely the features that attracted Chōei. The potato was pioneered as a famine relief measure in Ireland, with other European countries following suit. Scotland grew potatoes in response to famine in the 1740s, and the British government actively encouraged the growth of potatoes in 1795–96, as did Frederick the Great in Germany in 1745. It was not really until the end of the eighteenth century that a decline in the quality of varieties grown and increasing problems with disease broke the "potato utopia" spell. By this time in Ireland, potatoes already made up roughly 60 percent of the nation's food supply, and many of the poor relied upon them entirely for their sustenance. They had nothing, therefore, to fall back upon when potato blight devastated the crop.[63] Relying on the Dutch books that trickled through the port of Nagasaki for his information, Chōei could not have known that, at the same time on the other side of the world, potato-dependent Ireland was slipping toward a devastating famine.

Despite Chōei's efforts, potato consumption in Japan increased only slowly. In Hokkaido, which is now Japan's main center for their cultivation, potatoes were introduced from Russia in the eighteenth century and were encouraged by the shogunal government in land reclamation schemes late in the Edo period. Cultivation on a large scale began in the Meiji period after 1868, and potatoes now form the largest proportion of all tuber crops grown in Japan.[64]

---

61. Literally, "eight *shō* (= 1.8 liters) tuber." Eight was considered to be a lucky number.

62. Appendix A, pp. 190–91.

63. Bourke, *"Visitation of God"?*, pp. 11–14, 52.

64. Kodansha, ed., *Kodansha Encyclopedia of Japan*, 6: 231; Heibonsha, ed., *Nihonshi daijiten*, 3: 1046. The promise with which the white potato was viewed in the early twentieth century may also be seen in *Outlines of Agriculture*.

Buckwheat

The particular type of buckwheat that Chōei recommended in *Treatise on Two Things for the Relief of Famine* is described as a rapidly maturing crop that grows bigger and is more resistant to cold than regular buckwheat. This is much more difficult to identify than the potato, which is helpfully illustrated in the pamphlet in exquisite detail by Watanabe Kazan.[65] Chōei himself wrote that he was unsure of where the first of these buckwheat seeds came from. He called the buckwheat *hayasoba* (quick buckwheat), *sandosoba* (three-times buckwheat, because it matured three times a year), or *Sōteisoba*, after his friend the physician Fukuda Sōtei, who gave it to him.

Buckwheat is native to the Himalayas and has been grown in Japan since early times. It is of the same botanical type, *Fagopyrum esculentum*, as the common buckwheat known today. There are, however, several variations within the same type, such as summer and autumn varieties, and a notch-seeded buckwheat, in which the edges of the hull extend to form wings. Chōei believed this last type to be the one grown in Siberia and expressed regret that seeds were not available in Japan, because it could perhaps be harvested more frequently in a warmer climate. However, the Siberian type would more likely be *Fagopyrum tataricum*, or Tartary buckwheat. This actually belongs to a different species, and is a hardier but poorer plant. As a tentative conclusion, it seems probable that Sōtei had come across a variety of *Fagopyrum esculentum*, rather than some kind of new and better Western variety. From the description given, it can be inferred that it was a summer variety, which may help to explain why it grew both bigger and faster.[66]

Chōei's confusion about the type of buckwheat grown in Siberia is relatively understandable, considering that the source of his information was probably a Dutch book. The reason for other

---

65. See Fig. 1, pp. 192–93.

66. Makino, *Shin Nihon shokubutsu zukan*; De Candolle, *Origin of Cultivated Plants*; Simmonds, ed., *Evolution of Crop Plants*. I am grateful to Beatrice Bodart-Bailey for helping me to formulate this hypothesis.

mistakes is much less clear. For instance, when describing a place in Friesland, Holland, a topic presumably much more familiar to the Dutch or West European writers than Siberian agriculture, Chōei says it is a very mountainous place where the cold is extremely severe, and where nothing can grow except the aforementioned buckwheat. Perhaps the place he read about was not in Friesland at all, or perhaps he misinterpreted what he did read about Friesland. Mistakes such as these help to serve as a reminder of the enormous physical and linguistic boundaries that Chōei and the physicians were attempting to cross. In any case, the error does not seriously detract from his argument that there were cold and mountainous regions in the world where this crop had proved to be useful.

Incidentally, Chōei's view of Europe as a cold and inhospitable place seems to have been reflective of the general understanding at the time. Watanabe Kazan, too, wrote that the countries of Europe had been troubled by famine and cold until they overcame such problems through cultural advancement.[67] The National Learning scholar Hirata Atsutane surmised that the main reason Europeans roamed the world looking for trading partners was because, unlike the Japanese, they did not have sufficient resources at home.[68]

Malnutrition, Disease, and
Methods of Avoiding Epidemic Diseases

In considering further why Chōei and the Kōzuke physicians became interested in growing new crops as a weapon against famine, it is worth remembering that all of them grew up in rural areas, close to the farmers who were affected by the elements, for better or worse, every day of their lives. Chōei's birthplace of Mizusawa was in the north of Japan, where rice cultivation was hampered by the cold climate. Similarly, the mountainous regions of Kōzuke

---

67. Watanabe Kazan. "Gaikoku jijōsho," p. 19.
68. Hirata Atsutane, "Kodō taii," p. 143. In English, see also Keene, *The Japanese Discovery of Europe*. Atsutane was influenced by the observation made by Engelbert Kaempfer that Japan was a country with a mild climate and blessed with natural resources.

were not suited to growing rice, and it was natural for the Kōzuke farmer-physicians to experiment with other crops. Sōtei was even inspired to write a series of "buckwheat poems" and send them to his teacher.[69] *Treatise on Two Things for the Relief of Famine* provides further clues. In the following passage, Chōei shows sympathy for the workers on the land but is at once aware of the larger scale of the problem, including the consequences of malnutrition on the health of the populace:

Ah, how the farmers give their energies to farming! Although showered with rain and combed by the wind, irritated by sweat and the oil on their skins all dried up, they work untiringly and look forward to the harvest, only to meet with such disaster and have their efforts evaporate all at once. How can one not feel sorry for them? Accordingly, such a great calamity is not just that of the farmers, but of society at large. Even though these are prosperous times now and there are few who starve to death, if the price of rice jumps, then a day's work is not enough to buy a day's food. With regard to this matter, in desolate villages and cold hamlets, it comes to scraping the bark from trees or washing the muddy earth to eat. By doing so people are able to ward off starvation for a time, but because such foods are unusual, within one or two, or perhaps three or four months, there are many who fall ill and die. This is the reason why there is much sickness after a poor harvest. I am always worried by this.[70]

Chōei continued with this theme in the second pamphlet, *Methods of Avoiding Epidemic Diseases*. This was based, Chōei explained, on a preliminary discussion of epidemic diseases that he had written in a book called *On'ekikō* (Treatise on contagious diseases). He entrusted the revision and simplification of this medical work to Takahashi Keisaku. At the time, Keisaku was in Edo, as the head student at Chōei's school.

The pamphlet begins with a preface, in which Chōei described the synchronous relationship between epidemic diseases and famine, and the need for a method not only of treating epidemic diseases but of preventing them. He explained that, in order to facilitate people's thorough understanding, he wrote in Japanese rather than Chinese, the language of the literati.

---

69. Kanai, "Fukuda Kōsai no rangaku no michi to Agatsuma rangaku," p. 39.
70. Appendix A, pp. 183–84.

Methods of Avoiding Epidemic Diseases begins with an outline of methods of preventing epidemic diseases. In this, Chōei explained the dangers of poisonous atmospheres and the importance of caring for the digestive system through regular purging. This is followed by sections on hygienic practices for those caring for or visiting patients with epidemic diseases; what to do after people have died; information on preparing drugs; and finally a section on practical treatments for the sick.

The discussion below is an attempt to analyze these methods and treatments in order to gain an understanding of the process by which *ranpō* physicians introduced Western elements into their medical treatments and used them in conjunction with more traditional therapies. In order to do this, it will be necessary to ask to what extent it is possible to view such treatments as "Western" or "Chinese" in nature. It should be emphasized that the aim of this is not to judge how "progressive" the Japanese physicians were but to describe the practical manner in which they adopted and applied knowledge.

One of the most striking aspects of *Methods of Avoiding Epidemic Diseases* is the emphasis placed on preventive medicine. Another important feature in Chōei's writing is the idea of poisonous vapors present in the environment that are thought to be responsible for causing disease:

Essentially at times when epidemic fevers are rampant, they occur because there is a different kind of bad air[71] in the land; so that there are times when even if one is not infected immediately as a result of visiting someone sick, one can unintentionally be exposed to this atmosphere and spontaneously develop the disease. For this reason, people should take care of their bodies in order not to catch the disease.[72]

Chōei wrote that there were many fevers in rural areas because the front of the courtyard was not cleaned properly and the rooms

---

71. *Reiki* 戾気. I have interpreted this unusual compound as an alternative reading for 癘気, meaning a bad air that causes tropical diseases, etc. In addition, Chōei used several other expressions to refer to "bad air" including "gloomy air" (気の鬱する), "dirty air" (汚気), and "poisonous air" (毒気).

72. Appendix B, p. 200.

were gloomy. "Even if there were no poisonous fever in the first place, it spontaneously develops there," he stated.[73] He also emphasized the importance of adequate ventilation:

According to the customs of our country, not only with regard to epidemic fevers, but also in general, when we have a feverish illness we use heavy bedclothes and shut the window tight, or we place a screen around in order to keep out any draft. However, to think it is a good thing to do nothing but sweat is a terrible mistake.[74]

By implicitly setting the customs of his own country against those of another, Chōei appears to have obtained his information from foreign sources. However, similar concepts, thought of broadly as "miasmatic," were employed in both Chinese and Western medical thought at this time.

As described in the Introduction, traditional Chinese medical thought was based on a complex system in which the human body was seen to be a microcosm of the universe. The universe was in constant motion, and operated according to cyclic relationships that were influenced by the "five evolutionary phases," yin and yang, types of energy such as *qi* (*ki* in Japanese),[75] the calendar, and seasons. When the delicate balance among the elements in the system was disrupted, excesses or deficiencies in energy were created, and disease occurred. There were many reasons for the body to become imbalanced, for it was constantly barraged by disruptive influences known as *xie* (or *ja* in Japanese),[76] the meaning of which can be literally translated as "harmful emanations," "miasmas," or "evils."[77] These influences could be external, such as seasonal and epidemic diseases or climatic changes, or internal, such as imbalances of the emotions. Sometimes Tokugawa physicians referred to particular kinds of bad influences, such as "wind *ja*" or "cold *ja*."[78] So there was certainly a place for the idea that pathogenic agents

---

73. Appendix B, p. 202.

74. Appendix B, p. 202.

75. 気.

76. 邪.

77. Ozaki, "Conceptual Changes," p. 34. Porkert translates the term as "heteropathies." Porkert, *Theoretical Foundations of Chinese Medicine*, p. 52.

78. Ozaki, "Conceptual Changes," p. 35.

caused disease, but their effects were interpreted as forming part of a "pattern of causes leading to disharmony."[79] The entire system of Chinese medical thought was based on an intimate correlation between the human body and cosmological, environmental, and psychological factors.

Similarly, in the West, the ancient Hippocratic idea that "airs, waters, and places" affected the state of health was very influential. In the seventeenth and eighteenth centuries, there was a renewed interest in the environment, and particularly in bad smells, as a source of disease. It was a time when doctors became interested in connecting Galenic humoral theory, with its ideas of imbalances and predisposition to disease, with Hippocratic ideas about environmental and atmospheric influences.[80] Even in nineteenth-century Europe and America, the body continued to be seen "metaphorically as a system of dynamic interactions with its environment."[81] Thus, even if Chōei was being inspired to write by the latest he had read on Western theories of disease and epidemics, it was an easy task to equate concepts such as miasma with traditional Chinese ideas.

It has been suggested that Chinese physicians could have been influenced by Western miasmatic theorists. Chinese physicians in the nineteenth century, for example, promoted "foreign" methods such as cooling down underneath a tree or by a lake, or a "new" method of isolating plague victims. The idea of contagion, however, with the implication that the source of illness was within the body, was foreign to Chinese traditions, and isolation was not seriously advocated.[82] The absence of the idea of contagion in China was arguably the reason for major differences between public health policy in Europe, where quarantines were enforced, and that in China, where they were not.[83] Chōei, on the other hand, wrote of the need to isolate patients in hospitals, so that they might simultaneously receive better care and prevent the spread of

---

79. Lock, *East Asian Medicine*, p. 38.
80. Dobson, *Contours of Death*, p. 10.
81. Rosenberg, "Therapeutic Revolution," p. 487.
82. Benedict, *Bubonic Plague*, p. 109.
83. Ibid., p. 130.

infection. He pointed to the successful prevention of smallpox in some areas of Japan through the isolation of victims. At the same time, he was also aware of humanitarian concerns and urged people not to abandon their loved ones out of fear. His apparently inconsistent attitude to the relationship between bad air and contagion was probably not as strange as it first might seem. Contagionist and anticontagionist miasmatic explanations were not necessarily mutually exclusive, and environmental factors such as adequate ventilation could be important in both.[84]

There is one particularly interesting question raised by *Methods of Avoiding Epidemic Diseases* about the conception of death at the time. In the section about procedures for burial of the victims of disease, Chōei wrote: "When a patient dies from an epidemic fever, the body should be quickly prepared and buried. However, people who die from epidemic fever sometimes come back to life when they are exposed to the vapors of the earth; so be well aware of this and continue to watch out even after burial."[85] It was commonly believed that for a period shortly after the time of death, the spirit had not yet completely separated from the body and remained close by. Sometimes the name of the deceased was chanted in order to try to bring him or her back.[86] According to this interpretation, perhaps the idea of someone coming back to life was entirely reasonable.

In some Chinese theories, pestilential *qi* was believed to be an "earthly" *qi* rather than an atmospheric one, but whether these theories could have influenced Chōei's ideas about burial is unclear. Another suggestion is that the notion of coming back to life could somehow be related to the kind of idea expressed in a Chinese book of 1895 called *Shuyi yuebian* (Compilation on plague). According to this story, a man who was taken for dead and was about to be closed up in his coffin was saved by a thief who stole his burial clothes in the night, because their removal exposed him to cooling

---

84. Hamlin, "Predisposing Causes and Public Health in Early Nineteenth-Century Medical Thought," pp. 48–49.

85. Appendix B, p. 205.

86. Kodansha, ed., *Kodansha Encyclopedia of Japan*, 2: 80.

breezes, which brought about his recovery.[87] Of course, Chōei's writing predated this book, but the stories expressed in the Chinese work may not necessarily have been new. Western writers, on the other hand, appear to have been more concerned about the continuing damage the dead might do to the living through problems of putrefaction and harmful miasmas generated by overcrowded burial grounds. There was a movement during the eighteenth century in several European countries to have burials conducted outside the limits of towns and cities.[88]

It was important for Chōei, whether he had understood the European books on their own terms or not, to put new information into a form in which it could be readily accepted and understood. As Margaret Lock has observed in a discussion of medical systems and medical context, medical theory is culture-bound because "the questions raised by theoreticians and the methods used to answer them are products of a particular period in history."[89] Even if medical ideas and practices are introduced into a particular society, it is very difficult to introduce the social and cultural context of the new medical system at the same time. Although an individual doctor who has studied abroad "may change his beliefs radically . . . the system in which he must practice and the attitudes of patients will be important limiting factors on rapid changes in meaning associated with health and illness."[90] Similarly, nineteenth-century physicians in America were reluctant to part with traditional therapeutics even after they had been exposed to new ideas such as disease specificity, which undermined the traditional view of therapeutics and the body. This was because they still had to satisfy the demands of the patient in the traditional doctor-patient relationship.[91]

In practical terms, new treatments were implemented only very slowly, and this is reflected also in Chōei's document. Although doctors such as Chōei called themselves "physicians of Dutch

---

87. Benedict, *Bubonic Plague*, p. 108.
88. Riley, *The Eighteenth-Century Campaign to Avoid Disease*, pp. 100–110.
89. Lock, *East Asian Medicine*, p. 11.
90. Ibid., p. 12.
91. Rosenberg, "Therapeutic Revolution," pp. 497–504.

medicine," most of the medicines mentioned in the text were herbs that can be identified in books of traditional Chinese *materia medica*.

In *Methods of Avoiding Epidemic Diseases*, an emphasis is placed on emetic and purgative medicines and on sweating. These treatments were probably based on ideas in Japanese schools of Chinese medicine, which attached importance to eliminating stoppage or stagnation in the body. Such ideas were as common in Western medicine as they were in that of China, where the concept of balance encouraged the use of purgatives, emetics, sweating, and bleeding.

Innovations within Confucian medicine in Japan created a theoretical basis for the acceptance of Western medicine; in particular, an increasing interest in empiricism and the idea that medicine must be based on a thorough understanding of anatomy. The intellectual basis for *ranpō* medicine was prepared by changing the nature of traditional Confucian medicine in such a way that it was no longer antagonistic to Western thought.[92] Ozaki has proposed that this was the reason that people from many different intellectual backgrounds were able readily to take up *ranpō* medicine.[93] Certainly, the way the Kōzuke physicians became interested in Western medicine, even though their training was Chinese, appears to corroborate this. Both Fukuda Sōtei and Takahashi Keisaku studied with physicians trained in the *koihō* school of Chinese medicine. The *koihō* school, which "rejected the theoretical entities of Chinese medicine and undertook an empirical approach to clinical treatment," has also been noted for its role in easing the way for Western medicine in Japan.[94]

The changes that occurred in Japanese medicine during the Tokugawa period were the result of a long, slow process of reception and adaptation in response to both internal and external factors. Chōei and the Kōzuke physicians were practicing a kind of hybrid medicine that combined elements of both Western and

---

92. Ozaki, "Conceptual Changes," p. 233.
93. Ibid., p. 238.
94. Nakayama, "Ways of Thinking of Japanese Physicians," pp. 9–12.

Chinese traditions. They were able to do this because some schools of Chinese medicine in Japan had already divorced themselves from the traditional Chinese theoretical aspects that were incompatible with Western ideas. Furthermore, the similarity of the traditional concept of the body and therapeutics in Western and Asian medical systems of the time facilitated their hybridization.

Readership

For whom were Chōei's pamphlets intended? The question of readership is always a difficult one, linked inevitably to questions of literacy. Although literacy levels in Edo period Japan are believed to have been very high,[95] one must also address the question of what kinds of materials people at different levels of society were interested in reading. It was not the lowest echelons of society at which these pamphlets were aimed but those wealthier farmers and physicians who had the capacity to transmit such information. Indirectly at least, some sort of official attention was also probably desired.

In the preface to *Methods of Avoiding Epidemic Diseases*, Chōei wrote: "Although this is too insignificant and trifling a composition to be given an audience, if people are thereby able to escape such suffering, surely this project may be of some benefit to society."[96] Chōei's intentions are clear even through the veil of conventional modesty. Similarly, in *Treatise on Two Things for the Relief of Famine*, he emphasized the wide-reaching benefits of growing new crops as opposed to the limitations of building storehouses of grain, quoting a colleague as saying: "This is a fine and virtuous plan which should reach the whole land for all time."[97] In order to have such plans implemented far and wide, Chōei and his colleagues needed readers.

Some clues as to how they went about reaching these readers may be seen in the connections Chōei made through the Shōshikai study group in Edo. As noted above, the members of the Shōshi-

---

95. Moriya, "Urban Networks and Information Networks," pp. 118–23.
96. Appendix B, p. 199.
97. Appendix A, p. 185.

kai were vitally interested in the problems of famine relief and may well have provided some of the impetus for Chōei and his friends to engage in the writing of these works in the first place. Some evidence of the way in which Chōei was supported by the Shōshikai comes in the form of the botanical illustration of the potato plant for *Treatise on Two Things for the Relief of Famine*, drawn by Chōei's mentor Watanabe Kazan. In addition, *Methods of Avoiding Epidemic Diseases* contained a brief afterword, written by a man called Hagura, which praised the content and aims of the work. Since Watanabe Kazan maintained a friendship with an influential scholar called Hagura Geki, it is reasonable to assume it was he who had been asked to supply the afterword. Hagura served as the government intendant of several provinces in the Kantō region, including Kōzuke, and was therefore a Bakufu official of some status. He was later employed by the Senior Councilor (*rōjū*) Mizuno Tadakuni in the Tenpō Reforms.[98]

It can be assumed that having a man such as Hagura write the afterword to the pamphlet would have greatly increased both the document's credibility and its chances of being noticed by important government officials. Indeed, it was increasingly common for the work of unknown authors to carry the recommendation of a more prominent person.[99] Although it is questionable whether Chōei could be described in 1836 as an "unknown" (having published his ground-breaking *Fundamentals of Western Medicine* in 1832), he was in social terms merely a "town doctor" and was presumably in need of some helpful introductions to those in authority. A man such as Hagura with his Bakufu connections was of no small importance to Chōei. An official audience was desirable in terms of both influencing policymaking and enhancing his status if the works were well received. Since the government had previously been encouraged to promote the cultivation of sweet potatoes, perhaps Chōei had good reason to think that officials might do the same for his potato.

---

98. Satō, *Yōgakushi kenkyū josetsu*, p. 197.
99. Kornicki, *The Book in Japan*, p. 188.

Overtly at least, the pamphlets seem to be concerned with educating the ordinary public in order that they may help themselves. *Methods of Avoiding Epidemic Diseases*, in particular, was aimed at commoners. As we have seen, Chōei stated in the document that he wrote in Japanese rather than Chinese so as to facilitate understanding and that he recommended only medicines that could be used by lay people without harm. It was not unknown for works of this genre to be distributed to commoners and officials alike. Takebe Seian, discussed above for his role in writing about famine, is said to have presented his *Minkan bikōroku* to domain leaders in 1756, but, unable to wait for their official instruction, he made several copies and distributed them in rural areas.[100]

Gaining official permission to publish a book in the Edo period was a complicated procedure. It was very beneficial if novice authors cultivated contact with someone who was well informed of the many obstacles. Farmer-authors who wanted to publish their farm manuals, for example, cultivated contacts with the scholar Hirata Atsutane, who used his many connections throughout the country to help the farmers disseminate their books as widely as possible. In turn, Atsutane used the farm manuals as a way of promoting his theology in rural circles.[101] Although the case of Chōei and the Kōzuke physicians is a little different, because Chōei shared a significant responsibility for the authorship of the works, it is possible to imagine that they shared a similar relationship.

Some of the information contained in the two pamphlets suggests that it may have been intended to be transmitted by physicians or wealthy farmers, such as Chōei's students themselves. There is evidence that Chōei wrote to Harazawa Yoshimichi, a respected and wealthy physician from Noda, and sent him several copies of *Treatise on Two Things for the Relief of Famine*, asking him to distribute them among his acquaintances.[102]

---

100. Shirasugi, "Nihon ni okeru kyūkōsho no seiritsu to sono engen," p. 144.

101. Robertson, "Sexy Rice: Plant Gender, Farm Manuals, and Grass-Roots Nativism," pp. 253–54.

102. Letter quoted in Maruyama, *Gunma no ishi*, p. 89.

Many of the instructions in *Methods of Avoiding Epidemic Diseases* dealt with simple things such as ventilation and general cleanliness, which the average householder could easily understand and carry out. Humanitarian concerns, such as the importance of not being afraid to stay and care for sick loved ones, were also emphasized. There were also detailed descriptions of the preparation and uses of medicine, including Western medicines such as white soap from Holland, saffron, and ipecacuanha. Although large quantities of drugs—saffron, for example—were imported through Nagasaki,[103] there is some doubt as to whether they were readily available in rural communities. Chōei himself admitted this, for in the text he sometimes suggested alternatives to be used instead of these drugs in places where they could not be obtained. One of the procedures described was the distillation of sulfuric acid, which required a full day's work. Even if they had the necessary equipment, one must ask whether ordinary commoners would have had the time and energy to make a preparation such as this. Perhaps Chōei wished to encourage some industrious wealthy entrepreneur (of which there were many, physicians included) to produce and market it.

In many cases, then, the procedures described in *Methods of Avoiding Epidemic Diseases* make more sense if thought of as being transmitted by physicians to those they were designed to assist. Similarly, it was probably those educated farmers who had the economic capacity and the courage to plant new crops who would have been most interested in a work such as *Treatise on Two Things for the Relief of Famine*. Certainly Keisaku practiced what he preached; there is evidence in his diary that he was still planting Sōtei's "three times buckwheat" in 1872.[104] Presumably, the seeds for these plants would have been rather expensive if not yet readily available. Hence, even if Chōei and the physicians planned to distribute seeds, without official support their capacity to do so would have been limited. So they looked to encourage wealthy

---

103. Chaiklin, *Cultural Commerce and Dutch Commercial Culture*, p. 178. Chaiklin lists, for example, the following items in 1837: 900 taels ginseng, 65 taels saffron, 112.5 taels magnesia, 70 taels Berlin blue, 10 taels *radix ipecac*, 15 taels antimony, 8 taels Peruvian balsam.

104. Kanai, *Takahashi Keisaku nikki*, p. 459 (1872.4.16).

farmers to join in their plan, hoping to attract them perhaps as much from a desire for personal profit as out of humanitarianism.

In *Methods of Avoiding Epidemic Diseases*, one thing in particular stands out as an indication of the kind of people Chōei was trying to reach. In writing of the best method for preventing epidemic diseases, Chōei described the setting up of an isolation ward funded by wealthy merchants, farmers, and powerful persons in a "certain faraway country."[105] Chōei saw this as an important way of preventing the spread of disease. He related it to instances in his own country where smallpox cases had been isolated and suggested that this was the reason there were some places now free from smallpox. In writing of the importance and need for hospitals, Chōei can only have been trying to mobilize those who had enough power or money to set them up.

Finally, perhaps the excursion of Chōei and the Kōzuke physicians into the field of famine literature can be seen as a kind of preliminary professionalization strategy.[106] Although it is questionable to what extent physicians as a whole regarded themselves as a coherent group, and there was as yet no sign of a code of ethics or calls for registration, scholars of Western learning seem to have had a strong sense of identity. They linked their families through marriage and adoption. They attempted to demonstrate the value of Western learning through the practical application of new knowledge (to which they had exclusive access through their mastery of the Dutch language) to distressing social problems such as famine and epidemics. Their attempts to gain both popular and official acceptance of their publications can be seen as a desire for recognition: not merely in personal terms, but of the worth of their scholarly realm.

---

105. Appendix B, p. 205.

106. Douglas Klegon has described the process of professionalization along two dynamics: the first, the internal dynamic, refers to the efforts of practitioners to raise their status, define their special services, and achieve and maintain autonomy and influence through various strategies; the external dynamic refers to the relationship of an occupation to arrangements of power and the way in which this relationship affects the social meaning of an occupation. Klegon, "The Sociology of Professions: An Emerging Perspective," especially pp. 268–69, 271.

CHAPTER 4

"The Way of Medicine": Takahashi Keisaku's Daily Work

Takahashi Keisaku (1799–1875), of Yokō village near Nakanojō, was the youngest of the three Kōzuke physicians. Although he was Chōei's senior by five years, he outlived his ill-fated teacher by 25 years. Apart from the time he spent in Chōei's school in Edo during the early 1830s, Keisaku chose to live his long life quietly in Kōzuke. The following study of his activities provides a portrait of the daily work of a country doctor in the late Edo period. In particular, it demonstrates that Keisaku had many other duties apart from those of a medical doctor and that these diverse roles had a great influence on the conduct of his medical practice. The chapter also gives an indication of the expanse of Keisaku's personal networks. His constant stream of visitors and varied social life suggest that this was an important part of the way that medical, technological, and other information came to reach the mountains of provincial Kōzuke.

A *Gōnō* Physician

Keisaku sometimes signed his aesthetic works with the sobriquet *hannō*, meaning "semi-farmer." In fact, an examination of his diary quickly reveals that it is very difficult to separate the multiple roles he played in his community as farmer, doctor, village official, and poet. During certain periods of his life, such as the year he served as village headman, one role was allowed to dominate his work almost completely. Most of the time, however, he worked here and there according to demand.

As a farmer, Keisaku possessed land with an assessed yield of 11 *koku*.[1] He was not the richest person in the village, nor was a holding of this size especially large, but as one of only five landholders who had more than 10 *koku*, he was unquestionably among the village elite. His income also seems to have been substantially enhanced by silk farming; in the most profitable year, 1860, he sold his cocoons to a local merchant for as much as 15 *ryō* (1860.6.8).[2]

Keisaku appears to have done only a little of the farm labor himself; this fell mainly to his sons and to the women of the household. Many of his projects, including his period of study in Edo during the early 1830s and the brief establishment of a secondary medical practice in Maebashi, were possible only because he was free from the daily working of the farm. Indeed, one is struck by the apparent freedom of his lifestyle; he was frequently absent from home on medical business and on pleasure outings such as drinking and poetry parties. Keisaku's successive wives and his daughter-in-law Kise played a central role in supporting such a lifestyle. Even in 1873, when the household consisted of an aged Keisaku, Kise, her seventeen-year-old daughter Riya, and her two sons aged fourteen and eleven, the family still managed to record a harvest worth fifteen *ryō*. The crops included barley, soybeans, millet, glutinous and regular rice, red beans, wheat, and silk thread (1874.11.20). During the busiest times, other relatives and some wage laborers, both men and women, were employed. Similarly, after the death of his second wife, Keisaku arranged for the wife of his friend Yanagida Teizō to find him a housekeeper. This woman, who remained with Keisaku for some time, is referred to in the diary only as the "Echigo-baba" (old woman from Echigo) (1855.9.15).

----

1. Kanai, *Takahashi Keisaku nikki*, p. 602. A *koku* is generally considered to be equivalent to 4.96 bushels of rice. See also p. 31.

2. All references to the diary text in this chapter come from Kanai, *Takahashi Keisaku nikki*. References to the text take the form (year.month.day[s]). "Inter" is short for "the intercalary month of."

As a member of the local elite, Keisaku was involved in the tax affairs of the village, sorting out the return of loans, serving as a mediator in local disputes, and similar activities. He served as village headman for one year only, in 1857. In 1862, he asked to be relieved of his other official duties and passed his responsibilities to his son Keisuke, although he continued to be deeply involved in village affairs.

Keisaku did keep a careful eye on the agricultural work, especially on the silk farming, and recorded in his diary the various crops planted and harvested. For silk farming at least, this was typical practice. Work was generally carried out by women and supervised by the male household head.[3] As a highly educated member of the rural elite who experimented successfully in sericulture, Keisaku was a typical example of his *gōnō* (wealthy farmer) class. He recorded his silk-raising techniques in painstaking detail, bought silkworm egg cards and some of his mulberry leaves, and raised both spring and summer crops of worms. This kind of meticulous approach, taken by many Japanese silk farmers during the Edo period, has been described as an important factor in developing an intellectual framework for technological experimentation.[4] It remains to be seen in this chapter whether the same may be said for wealthy rural physicians in their approach to medicine.

The Diary

Keisaku's diary stretched over 36 years of the latter part of his life, from 1838 until 1874. Amounting to more than 500 printed pages, it was published in 1995 through the efforts of his descendant Takahashi Tadao and a local historian, Kanai Kōsaku. The diary is a concise record of Keisaku's daily activities, medical visits, visitors, and the workings of his farm. It also contains detailed observations of the economic market and some current affairs. On the back cover of one of the volumes, he wrote "this diary should

---

3. Morris-Suzuki, "Sericulture and the Origins of Japanese Industrialization," p. 112.
    4. Ibid., p. 121.

never be lost," which indicates something of the importance he attached to it.[5]

On the whole, the daily entries of the diary were kept remarkably faithfully, but there were also several large gaps in the record over its 36-year course. Each of these lapses, which occurred in the years 1840–52, 1859, and 1866, appears to have been associated with traumatic events in Keisaku's life. For example, although there is no overt mention of the event in the text itself, the final entry in 1839 came just six days after Takano Chōei was sentenced to life in prison. When Keisaku finally picked up his brush again at the beginning of 1853, Chōei had been dead for about two years. He entitled the new volume "Silk Farming Diary," and there is little evidence of medical activity. His concise style is particularly prominent at this time, as demonstrated by the first few entries:

1st Month
1st day   Fine. Cold.
2nd day   Warm.
3rd day   Ditto. My wife died at about ten in the morning.   (1853.1.1–3)

Sporadic entries continued for a month or so before settling down to a daily pattern. The next break came in 1858, following the death of his sister-in-law, Kono. The period surrounding her death, too, was marked by infrequent diary entries, followed by a two-week lapse and a fresh start in a new book. It was another five months before entries become regular and informative again. The following year of 1859 is also missing. Finally, the missing year of 1866 was one in which his youngest son Shirō died of illness. In other instances of the death of friends or relatives, too, the entries immediately following often contained only weather reports, even if the diary was not left off completely.

Thus, although Keisaku seldom expressed his emotions in the diary itself, his writing appears to have been an activity significantly connected to the way he felt. The decade of silence prompted by Chōei's arrest, in combination with the lack of medical activity following the recommencement of the diary in 1853,

---

5. Kanai, *Takahashi Keisaku nikki*, p. 246 (1861).

and the consequent emphasis on silk farming, would seem to indicate that Chōei's fall from grace caused some kind of upheaval in Keisaku's life. The events of the *bansha no goku* may have discouraged him from practicing medicine, only to return to it after Chōei's death.[6] Whereas in the year of Chōei's arrest Keisaku made 145 medical visits, he made only eight in the year the diary recommenced. His eventual full return to medical practice is suggested by a record of 128 visits in 1855.

Even in 1873, nearly twenty years later, when doctors were required to submit their résumés to official inspection, Keisaku does not appear to have felt he could write the truth about his relationship with Chōei. He recorded in his diary the details that he planned to submit: that he began to study with Chōei in 1826, much earlier than he really did, and that he returned home in 1828, though Chōei was at this time still in Nagasaki (1873.7.8). It is likely that in so doing he was trying to distance himself from the period in which Chōei found himself in trouble. Several days after this entry, however, he complained that "due to the imprudence of the local authority" his résumé had not been passed on, and he was forced to rewrite it. Unfortunately, he gave no indication whether he chose to tell the truth the second time.

Medical Life

The average annual number of medical visits Keisaku made over the entire period of the diary was 126 visits on an average of 83 days per year.[7] The vast majority of visits were made in his own village of Yokō. Therefore, even taking into account the amount of time it took to travel from village to village on foot, this was far from a full-time occupation. The busiest year was 1862, in which Keisaku made a total of 432 visits in 156 days. Notably, this was a year in which Japan was hit by epidemics of measles and cholera, which are discussed in detail below. The smallest number of visits was made in 1853, the first year after the recommencement of the

---

6. This view is shared by the editors of Keisaku's diary, and Tabata Tsutomu in his article "Bakumatsu ni okeru ichi chihō ran'i no jiseki ni tsuite," pp. 45–58.

7. Kanai, *Takahashi Keisaku nikki*, p. 576.

diary. All but one of the visits in this year were made to his brother-in-law and friend, Nara Anpei.

Despite, or perhaps because of, the fact that there was not generally enough medical work to fill the days, when the diary opens in the fourth month of 1838, Keisaku had recently opened a secondary medical practice located in what is now the outskirts of Maebashi. Making an average of one medical visit per day, his enthusiasm bubbled over into the translation in his spare time of a Dutch book by ten Haaf (1720–91).[8] The secondary practice was, however, abortive; he returned home to Yokō village just four months later. This decision may well have been based on his own health, rather than the failure of the practice, for during his four months in Maebashi, he was plagued by an eye infection (apparently caught from a patient) that affected his ability to read and write and recurring bouts of fever, headache, and ague. This was followed by a severe stomach cramp shortly after his return, which prompted him to request treatment from his friend and neighbor Teizō (1838.7.30).

Keisaku's medical work consisted of a mixture of home visits, examinations performed upon request at his own house, and the simple dispensing of medicine. There were also instances in which he examined patients at the house of a third person. Severe cases or those in distant villages often involved an overnight stay, usually at the house of the patient. In other urgent cases, he sent his palanquin to fetch patients and bring them to stay with him (1857.9.8). Incidentally, Keisaku appears to have procured the palanquin,

---

8. Ten Haaf was a Dutch surgeon and lithotomist from Delft. The name of the book Keisaku translated was *Verhandeling over de voornaamste kwetzuuren, die den scheepsheel-meesteren op's Lands schepen van oorlog kunnen voorkomen; mitsgaders over het niet of al afzetten der leden* (Report on the most common injuries encountered by ship's surgeons on the nation's warships; together with amputation rates) and was published in Rotterdam in 1781. A copy of Keisaku's manuscript, which he entitled *Gunchū biyō* (Preparations for the battlefield), is held by the Kyoto University Medical Library and contains translations of the three chapters on bruises, gunshot wounds, and head wounds. See Miyashita, "A Bibliography of the Dutch Medical Books Translated into Japanese," p. 46. Another of ten Haaf's books was translated by Satō Taizen (1804–72). See Goodman, *Japan: The Dutch Experience*, p. 175.

which was an important status symbol as well as a practical item, in 1856 (7.22), the year after he returned to medical practice.

The name, sex, and native village of his patients were carefully recorded in diary entries. As one might expect of a country practice, there was a mixture of men, women, and children of all ages. After the initial visit, most patients required one or two follow-up visits, often made on a daily basis. In severe cases, Keisaku sometimes made as many as nine or ten visits.

Payments were not generally mentioned in the diary, but a separate record was discovered that detailed for one year only the medical problems of patients, the drugs used to treat them, and remuneration received. Since these cases do not overlap with those in any of the years in the diary, Kanai has suggested that this record may have been for one of the missing years of 1859 or 1866.[9] Of the 114 patients treated in the year, 65 made some form of monetary payment, which ranged from ten *hiki* to one *ryō*. It is not really possible to determine from the information presented by Kanai whether people paid according to the number of times they were visited, or according to the nature of the treatment, or whether they simply paid whatever they could afford. The highest payment of one *ryō* was from a woman treated for syphilis: a case in which Keisaku made a total of 70 visits. In the diary itself, Keisaku commonly recorded only end-of-year presents such as fish and rice wine. These tended to be from students rather than patients. On the other hand, people quite often brought a keg of wine when they requested a house call.

The separate record of visits is also a valuable source of information about the problems Keisaku treated, for in the diary itself he did not usually reveal the nature of his patients' illnesses. According to the medical record, the great majority of problems Keisaku dealt with were gastrointestinal disorders, with symptoms such as vomiting, diarrhea, and stomach pains. These were followed in number by syphilis and skin complaints, including scabies, and wounds. There were also fevers and chills and eye inflammations. Women's

---

9. Kanai's summary of this document is provided in the appendix to *Takahashi Keisaku nikki*, pp. 578–82.

disorders included morning sickness, cramps, and cracked nipples. Several of the syphilis patients were women. Worms, hemorrhoids, and urinary problems were also mentioned.

The drugs Keisaku used for treating these disorders were a mixture of herbs, imported medicines, and prepared medicines. In addition to common medicinal herbs such as peony, Chinese rhubarb, licorice, and bitter orange, some medicines were referred to by generalized names such as "stomach tonic" or "pills for protecting the soul." This suggests that they were probably prepared medicines, either mixed in advance by Keisaku himself or purchased. Several of these prepared medicines are listed in Keisaku's *Zuikōdō hōshū* (Collection of treatments at Zuikō's school).[10] It was not unusual for the prepared medicines to contain a combination of traditional and imported ingredients. For example, a "strengthening tonic" used a combination of cinchona, camphor, and bitter orange peel. Ipecacuanha was mixed with potassium tartrate (an emetic), flour, and sea onion for a purge. Other Western medicines Keisaku used were magnesia and jalap. Interestingly, in some instances he referred to drugs such as hollyhock and cinnamon by Western names (*alta* and *kaneel*, respectively, written in *katakana* script), while in others he referred to the same drugs by their Chinese characters. Did this depend on the source of his prescription? Or was he simply as comfortable with one name as with the other? In any case, his use of drugs as evidenced by these documents provides a firm indication of the "hybrid" nature of *ranpō* medicine in the late Edo period.

Those problems which Keisaku did mention in the diary itself are almost exclusively surgical cases, often the result of accidents. For example, he attended several instances of attempted suicide (1839.2.20, 1856.6.7, 1861.8.20. 1865.8.4), farming accidents caused by hatchets or sickles (1855.11.3, 1862.3.5), injuries sustained when falling from or being trampled by horses (1861.8.11, 1870.10.3), and a patient who fell from a tree (1867.9.8). He often recorded the administering of cupping treatments and the piercing of boils. Women with swellings on or in their breasts were another fre-

---

10. Takano Chōei Zenshū Kankō Kai, ed., *Takano Chōei zenshū*, 1: 245–63.

quent problem. Other common diseases to appear in the record were syphilis, smallpox, and eye infections. Not all surgical cases were due to accidents: Keisaku treated a relative who had her ear cut by a retreating robber (1861.12.12). He also attended a policeman who sustained injuries to the shoulder, arms, brow, and behind the ear when trying to arrest a member of a rebel group (*akutō*) in the turbulent year of the 1868 Restoration (1868.9.6). Presumably, the fact that he specifically mentioned the details of these cases meant that they were unusual or interesting to him, while the silent majority of intestinal disorders was too mundane to record.

Although childbirth was traditionally attended by midwives, Keisaku appears to have had at least some involvement in obstetrics. He was called to two difficult childbirths (1860.1.11, 1862.2.10) and on two occasions carried out an "operation" to remove the afterbirth (1855.1.5, 1870.6.4). In another instance, he dispensed a medicine to stimulate the discharge of the afterbirth rather than attending himself (1871.10.29). He was also present when his own daughter Kato was giving birth in 1863 (10.20). The baby was in the wrong position, and he called on a local doctor, Hayashi Kenryū, of Ōzuka village, to go with him and turn it around. He was required to remove the placenta in Kato's case too, which he did surgically "with a hook." Placing difficult births in the hands of male doctors and restricting the use of obstetric tools among midwives is often discussed as part of the medicalization of childbirth and the gradual monopolization by men of a traditionally female occupation. In Japan, the medicalization of childbirth began in the second half of the eighteenth century, accompanied by a growing interest in human anatomy and the development of obstetric instruments.[11] Keisaku's role in obstetrics provides an interesting example of the extent to which this process was under way in nineteenth-century rural Japan, not only for obstetricians but for ordinary practitioners too. This is an interesting point for two reasons. First, rural areas are usually thought to have been "backward," and the women who lived there reluctant to accept new practices. Second, because birth was traditionally thought to be "impure," female relatives

---

11. See, for example, Shinmura, *Shussan to seishokukan no rekishi.*

who assisted in the delivery were expected to observe a period of taboo.[12] Keisaku does not appear to have adhered to any such prescription, for he treated patients as usual the following day.[13] Keisaku's involvement in childbirth suggests that it was already beginning to be seen as a medical activity rather than a ritual, even in rural areas. This is an area ripe for further investigation.

At the same time as Kato was giving birth, Keisaku's daughter-in-law Kise, who was in the last month of pregnancy, had her waters break. She continued in this state, with no sign of labor pains, for the next five days. Keisaku became so worried about her that he wrote three *waka* poems and took one of them to the local Shinto shrine to pray. While he was yet to return, Kise finally gave birth, and he came home to find both mother and child doing well (1863.10.25). It is important to note that even as a doctor, he felt he could achieve more by devoting a poem to the shrine than by staying at the woman's bedside.

Keisaku does appear to have been circumspect about which cases he chose to take on. He was not above putting his own needs before those of his patients. There were times when he refused to make visits because of a hangover (1856.11.23), because he was drunk (1861.3.28), because he had a cold (1855.3.4), or because the road was too hard for his old legs (1863.9.15). Some cases were simply rescheduled for a more convenient time. Others were refused on medical grounds. For example, in 1856 he refused to visit a patient because the man "disliked his medicine and the treatment would be of no use" (1856.3.9). Sometimes there was simply nothing more he could do. In 1855, after treating a woman with an unspecified illness nine times over a period of two months, she appeared to be making no improvement, and he refused to make any further visits (4.15). This may have been in order to save face should she die.

---

12. Steger, "From Impurity to Hygiene: The Role of Midwives in the Modernisation of Japan," p. 177.

13. According to Shinmura, from the Insei and Kamakura periods, impurity was actually identified as beginning with the afterbirth; as long as a man left the room before the afterbirth was delivered, he would not be considered "polluted." This idea may have been operating here, or it may indicate that traditional attitudes to impurity were weakening.

Similarly, when called to treat an infant with an intestinal tumor or ulceration, he judged the condition to be already too critical to treat (1856.10.28). In other difficult cases, such as Kato's confinement above, it appears to have been quite common for the local doctors to call upon one another for help. No matter how sick they might become, close relatives, friends, or influential people were watched over until the very end.

As a doctor, and a man who lived to a remarkably old age in a medically precarious world, Keisaku was no stranger to death. Within the space of two years, he lost his first and second wives to illness. As noted above, his first wife Tsutako's death occurred at the very beginning of the 1853 "Silk Farming Diary," and her symptoms were not described. His second wife, Isako, appears to have suffered dreadful stomach pains before her death in 1855. Keisaku sent a messenger to call for Teizō, but by the time he was able to come, she had already died (1855.7.10). Shortly, the tables were turned, when Teizō fell gravely ill later the same year. Keisaku stayed at Teizō's bedside for four nights before he died. Two other doctors acquainted with Teizō were present too: one local and one who had made the journey from Shibukawa (1855.11.17–21).[14] Keisaku's devotion to Teizō and his family may be measured by the fact that, over the years, he was present at the deaths of his adopted son Teizō (II) in 1861 and eldest grandson Sachūta in 1865 and that he treated intensively his third grandson Asaburō (who was also his student) prior to his death in 1872. In his own family, Keisaku was forced to watch three of his five children die of illness.

Standing by, watching loved ones die, with so little in his power to help them, how did a doctor come to terms with his own inadequacies? Something of an answer may be found in a preface that Keisaku wrote for his student Yamamoto Taian in 1859.[15]

A person who practices medicine should recognize that to suffer illness is in the first nature of humans, and should treat others with a selfless sincerity and consideration. . . .

---

14. Kogure Sokuō (1789–1862). Kogure was a doctor and nativist scholar who studied medicine with Hanaoka Seishū and Takano Chōei.

15. This preface is reproduced in Kanai, *Takahashi Keisaku nikki*, pp. 183–84.

It is natural that people become sick, and natural that they recover. When a doctor gives people medicine, or uses various other skills to try to heal them, he is only assisting nature. . . . In medicine, there is only error, never success. To heal the various illnesses completely is to think deeply about and absorb the meaning of the power of nature. If, when all manner of medicines and skills have been exhausted to no effect, it means one's own thought has gone against the natural powers of nature, and this must be called medical error.

Thus, for Keisaku, medicine was subordinate to the healing processes of nature. It was "natural that people become sick, and natural that they recover." Presumably, it was also natural that some patients died, and in these cases, no matter what techniques the doctor might use, his efforts would be fruitless and errant. When seen in this light, the turning away of difficult cases appears less cold-hearted. Indeed, although family members, close friends, and influential people warranted a compassionate bedside presence until the very end, in many terminal cases the doctor could do little more for them than if he had turned them away.

This was also the traditional attitude in England, where, as Porter and Porter described, "Both medical theory and practice respected the fact that living and dying lay in Nature's hands, as the best Classical medicine stipulated, or were directed by Providence."[16] It was the duty of physicians only to make the prognosis of death, so that people could prepare themselves properly; after that they were not necessarily expected to attend the death. In the eighteenth century, however, there was a gradual change in the perception of the physician's role at the deathbed. Increasingly, he was expected to provide comfort, often in the form of pain relief through alcohol and opium, and to attend as a friend, when there was nothing more to be done. Death, too, was slowly becoming medicalized.[17]

Of course, not all illnesses were incurable, and the doctor was in demand. This was especially so during times of epidemic disease. In 1862, the Nakanojō region was hit by an epidemic. Keisaku first

---

16. Porter and Porter, *Patient's Progress*, p. 144.
17. Ibid., pp. 147–52.

identified the epidemic as an outbreak of measles (*mashin*). He was quick to note that many "foolish people" were dying from the overuse of medicines such as ginseng, poisonous snake, quinine, and saffron (6.26). By the middle of the next month, he found himself treating nine patients a day and recorded that the patients had diarrhea, collapsed, and died within twenty to thirty days.[18] He did note, however, that many patients who had the disease in combination with another medical problem or who used a "warming" medicine died, whereas only a few of those who used a "cooling" medicine did so (7.18). A close friend who succumbed to the disease displayed symptoms of sepsis and died within the space of five days (7.22–26).

Things went from bad to worse. At the beginning of the eighth month, prayers were being held to drive away the measles spirit. As the number of victims increased, Keisaku went from taking his favorite student, Gōsai, with him on his rounds to sending him in his place. He found he had to limit his visits to his own village in order to cope. Even so, he treated as many as eighteen patients in a day, lamenting the fact that instead of writing poetry, as he would have preferred, he had to spend the beautiful clear autumn nights in vain (8.15). During this period, he often did not return home until nine or ten o'clock at night. When the wife of his student Yamamoto Taian fell critically ill with the disease, Keisaku was forced to decline to attend her, much against his will, for the journey would take too long and mean neglecting patients closer to home (8.16). At the end of the eighth month, he included in his journal news of an outbreak of a severe epidemic disease in Edo and along the Nakasendō, in Maebashi and Kiryū. It was popularly called *korori*, though Keisaku was sure the disease must be scarlet fever.[19] He did not appear to relate this outbreak to the disease currently afflicting his community (8.30), but toward the end of the intercalary eighth month, someone from a nearby village died from *korori* disease (inter 8.21).

---

18. Diarrhea is common in severe cases of measles in places where it is accompanied by protein-calorie malnutrition, such as rural Africa. See Grist et al., *Diseases of Infection: An Illustrated Textbook.*

19. *Shōkōnetsu* 猩紅熱.

Keisaku's account of measles and the strange new *korori* disease is somewhat confusing. The word *korori* meant something like "suddenly" or "without resistance," and was used because of the alarming rapidity with which people succumbed to the disease. Later, when it was recognized as cholera, the term was used interchangeably with the word *korera*. In 1862, both measles and cholera were epidemic in Japan,[20] and it is quite possible that Keisaku's account is confused because the diseases were circulating at the same time.

Public Health and Vaccinations

Cholera was brought to Japan by foreign ships entering Nagasaki first in 1822 and then again in 1858. The second of these epidemics was very severe and spread the length of the country.[21] At this time, Keisaku recorded an official notice from Edo that suggested cinnamon, dried ginger root, and longan[22] as protection against the disease. So, as both a member of the village elite and a local doctor, it was he who received this official information and was responsible for its dissemination in order to protect the health of his local community. Cholera's frightening capacity to kill in the space of days encouraged all sorts of speculation about its cause. Many of these theories reflected resentment of the foreigners who brought the disease with them. For instance, Keisaku recorded rumors suggesting that someone had put poison in the Tamagawa River in Edo or that returning American ships had caused the disease by poisoning or doing a lot of washing in the sea (1858.8.15), and commented that the rumors were a bad sign of the times. In other instances, he was more scathing on the subject of people's ignorance. Another outbreak in 1874 prompted him to write: "Recently, many adults and children alike suffer from sudden abdominal pain, diarrhea, and vomiting. The children with severe cases can die within as little as a day and a night. This disease is popularly called *korori*, and it is said that if a sheet of red paper with the characters

20. See Jannetta, *Epidemics and Mortality.*
21. Ibid., pp. 155–72.
22. *Nephelium longana*, a plant related to the lychee.

for 'horse' and 'cow' written on it is hung outside the doorway, the disease will not come inside. What absurdity!" (1874.7.6).

The achievements of *ranpō* doctors in helping to bring Jennerian vaccinations against smallpox to Japan have often been noted. It is arguable that the dramatic results achieved by vaccination did much to encourage the wider acceptance of Western medicine, not only among private physicians but eventually by the shogunate itself.[23] As Ann Jannetta has indicated, the difficulties of obtaining vaccine and keeping it alive brought together groups of Japanese physicians who eventually created "a national network of physicians aligned with Western medicine." These networks, she continued, "became the professional networks that would successfully advance the cause of Western medicine in the Meiji era."[24] Even here, however, the principle of practicality reigned. As Beukers has argued, variolation and vaccination were "not accepted because they were theoretically better founded, they were accepted for their proven effectiveness."[25]

Although the exact scale of Keisaku's work is unclear, he too had a role to play in bringing vaccinations against smallpox to his community. The first instance of this in the diary occurred in 1860, when he obtained a vaccine through connections he had with a local poetess, Morita Kōgetsu. She brought the vaccine with her from her village of Iwamoto. With this, Keisaku vaccinated his granddaughter Riya, who was nearly three years old at the time (1860.inter 3.4). Twelve days later, the family held a celebration for the success of the vaccination. After thus confirming that the vaccine had taken, Keisaku vaccinated his ten-year-old grandson from the next village (1860.inter 3.21). Two days later, he returned the vaccine to Kōgetsu in Iwamoto.

---

23. See Beukers, "The Fight Against Smallpox in Japan: The Value of Western Medicine Proved," pp. 59–77. Chinese methods of variolation, in which a powder was made from the crusts of the sores of smallpox patients and was blown into the nostrils of children, had been known for some time in Japan, but were unpopular because they sometimes resulted in full-blown outbreaks of smallpox.

24. Jannetta, "The Introduction of Jennerian Vaccination in Nineteenth-Century Japan," p. 9.

25. Beukers, "The Fight Against Smallpox in Japan," p. 76.

Unfortunately, we do not know in what form this vaccine came. Since the easiest way to transport the fragile cowpox virus was on the arms of children who had recently been vaccinated, it is most likely that the vaccine used was in the form of lymph.[26] Perhaps this is why Keisaku obtained the vaccine through a female friend, so that she might accompany a small child carrying the virus.[27] Although Keisaku made no further record of other vaccinations at this time, given the difficulties of keeping the vaccine alive and the careful delay he made between the vaccination of one grandchild and the next, he probably intended to use the vaccine for the wider community. His developing interest in vaccination can be seen in the fact that his student Yamamoto Taian went to Edo in the eighth month of the following year (1861) for a period of around two months to study under Ōtsuki Shunsai at the Edo Vaccination Institute and obtain a vaccination license (1861.10.7).

In another entry, Keisaku visited a doctor in Nakanojō to obtain cowpox vaccine. With this, he attempted to vaccinate his two-year-old grandson, Matsusaburō, but the attempt failed (1864.4.27). Presumably, the vaccine had already lost its potency. Later, this doctor, Noguchi Ryōsuke, was ordered by the prefectural government to carry out extensive vaccinations on all children under the age of ten years in 1871 (3.6). This appears to have been the first instance in which the government in this region actually promoted vaccinations against smallpox, despite the fact that some domains had taken an active stance as early as 1849, when the cowpox vaccine first arrived in Japan.[28] In other parts of Kōzuke, Annaka domain took up vaccinations in 1856, and Maebashi in 1857.[29] Perhaps the Nakanojō region was hindered by the fact that it was *hatamoto* land and effectively under direct Bakufu rule. Even though the cowpox vaccine had reached many areas of Japan in the first year of its introduction, vaccinations did not gain the support of the

---

26. Jannetta, "The Introduction of Jennerian Vaccination," p. 7.

27. One of the entries suggests that she had a child with her, but the evidence is ambiguous.

28. Jannetta, "The Introduction of Jennerian Vaccination," pp. 8–9.

29. Maruyama, *Gunma no ishi*, p. 379.

Bakufu until 1858.[30] The Edo Vaccination Institute was made official only in 1860. An indication of the reluctance to embrace vaccination is that even the *hatamoto* overlord Tominaga lost two of his children, aged six and nine, to smallpox in 1857 (1.14).

On the other hand, it has been suggested that because of the limited rights that *hatamoto* had over their villages, their territories may actually have had more autonomy than elsewhere.[31] It is therefore difficult to explain why Keisaku, with his strong medical networks, took so long to promote vaccination in his village after his return to medical practice in 1855. Possibly he had been so badly frightened by the events of the *bansha no goku* in 1839 that he did not feel free to participate until the Bakufu government had given the procedure its full blessing.

Networks and Book-Lending

The logistics of keeping cowpox vaccine alive made it essential for regional doctors to cooperate. As we have seen in the example of Keisaku's poetess friend, even those from outside the medical arena were willing to help. These networks were established long before the discovery of vaccine. For example, the local doctors living in Nakanojō and its surroundings seem to have helped one another out on a regular basis. They called on their colleagues to assist with difficult treatments and often met at the houses of patients who could afford more than one doctor. Sometimes they lent one another equipment. In 1850, Keisaku received a letter from another doctor asking him to visit a certain patient. Since he was unable to attend himself, he lent the other doctor a catheter (6.13). Further evidence for the way doctors cooperated can be seen in a letter from Takahashi Kenji of Shibukawa to Mochizuki Shunsai of Nakanojō, in which Kenji apologized for administering medicine in Shunsai's absence, and asked him for his opinion of the treatment.[32]

---

30. Jannetta, "The Introduction of Jennerian Vaccination," p. 9.

31. Howell, "Social Disorder and Moral Reform in Late Tokugawa Japan" pp. 4–5.

32. Kanai, "Takano Chōei monka Nakanojōmachi Mochizuki Shunsai no hizō monjo o haiken shite," p. 24.

Keisaku often stayed the night at Teizō's house in Isemachi, sometimes returning home from parties there "well inebriated" (1839.10.30). He continued to visit and stay the night occasionally even after the death of his friend. With the addition of local pharmacist Negishi Shūzō, Keisaku and Teizō appear to have formed something of a threesome. They often boiled up ointments together at Shūzō's house, which was situated quite close to Teizō's in Isemachi (for example, 1839.10.25). It was without doubt a convenient location, for Shūzō was the proprietor of a combined drugstore and brewery: not only were the ingredients for the ointment close at hand, but the wine for parties afterward, too. All three participated in Takano Chōei's lecture series in 1833, and Shūzo's name also appears in Chōei's letters. Keisaku often exchanged books with Shūzō, whose reading interests extended to books on poetry, medicine, and calligraphy.

Indeed, one of the ways in which the doctors cemented their relationships was through the exchange of books. In the absence of public libraries, the private exchange of books in the Edo period was common practice.[33] Even with the advent of publishing, it was still common to copy complete books by hand, especially if they were rare.[34] There are numerous instances in Keisaku's diary in which he and his students copied the books they borrowed, especially those concerned with Western learning.

Keisaku kept a lending notebook between the years 1826–37 and again in 1845–48, in which he recorded the titles of the books he borrowed and lent, as well as the names of the people who borrowed them.[35] Later, he no longer kept a separate notebook but made entries in his diary noting when books were lent or returned. As might be expected, most of the identifiable borrowers of medical books were doctors (with the notable exception of an ascetic monk). Interestingly, it is largely the same group of names that appears against the titles of all kinds of other books, ranging from *waka* and *haikai* poetry collections to Confu-

---

33. Kornicki, *The Book in Japan*, p. 405.
34. Ibid., p. 243.
35. Kanai, *Takahashi Keisaku nikki*, pp. 525–32.

cian studies to Chinese poems to military and travel tales and
books about manners and customs. In the lending notebook there
is a marked drop in the number of medical books loaned after 1845,
which is probably a reflection of the period in which Keisaku
was not working as a doctor. One of the most frequent borrowers,
of both medical and other books, was Teizō. Keisaku borrowed
many books in return, including copies of the *Analects*, a military
biography, a book on gonorrhea, books of *waka* poems, and
many others.

If Keisaku did not buy his medicines from Shūzō, then he
bought them from the owner of another drugstore in Nakanojō,
Koitabashi Kensai (1798–1862). Kensai had been born into a priestly
family but handed his hereditary responsibility over to his younger
brother and became a doctor. After studying medicine under
Hanaoka Seishū, he returned home to run the pharmacy. Both
Kensai and his brother Yoshisato, who did become a Shinto priest,
exchanged books with Keisaku. Yoshisato, the priest, was interested in *kokugaku*, poetry, language, and orthography. In 1856, he
asked Keisaku to write out a copy of the Sanskrit alphabet for him.
It is a fine reflection of the level of Keisaku's skill as a calligrapher
that he was able to do so.

Kensai, the pharmacist, was interested in Western medical books
and *kokugaku*. By the nineteenth century, local intellectuals were
expected to have knowledge of both *kokugaku* and *rangaku*.[36] Both
schools of scholarship were influenced by the concept of *jitsugaku*,
or "practical learning,"[37] and it is perhaps this aspect, in addition to
the very strong influence of the Shinto faith in the local community, that attracted educated commoners such as Kensai and Keisaku. For example, in 1860, Kensai lent Keisaku a *kokugaku* book
written by Ōta Junzō (1816–62), a patriot who rejected the spread
of Western learning and called for a "holy way." This book appears
to have greatly impressed Keisaku with its "unshakeable opinions"
(1860.11.30).

---

36. Miyachi, *Bakumatsu ishinki no bunka to jōhō*, p. 23.
37. Aoki, *Zaison rangaku no kenkyū*, p. 77.

It is possible that Keisaku's interest in book lending was inspired by Itō Chūtai, his teacher of medicine from Shinano. He, too, appears to have had an extensive library and book-lending network. According to the research of Aoki Toshiyuki, many of the books in Chūtai's collection were handwritten manuscripts, for he was a diligent copyist. Although Chūtai was a doctor of *koihō* medicine, he was interested in Western medicine too and made copies of many Dutch books during a period in which he was working at Osaka castle.[38] Indeed, it was thanks to Chūtai's copy of Keisaku's notes that historians were able to learn of Takano Chōei's lecture series in 1833. As documented in Keisaku's notebook, the two also shared other books. Several books in their respective collections overlap, indicating that they may have been copied from one another. In addition, Chūtai appears to have been a frequent visitor at Teizō's house, where he made copies of Chōei's books. He recorded the fact that the books were Teizō's along with the date that he copied them in the back of at least two of these.[39] As for Chūtai's own book-lending network, Aoki cited at least one example of a doctor willing to pay Chūtai to borrow and copy his books.[40] The exchange of books between Chūtai and Keisaku demonstrates that book-lending was not limited to close-knit village circles, or even between Edo and individual villages, but was also developing interregional links in country areas. The links in this case were facilitated by a teacher-student relationship.

Keisaku was also visited at least once by a commercial booklender, which suggests that they were not merely a phenomenon of the cities, but were permeating rural areas too. On this occasion, he returned ten volumes of a well-known Chinese novel and borrowed another ten of the next series (1856.12.4).[41]

---

38. Ibid., pp. 192–93.
39. Ibid., pp. 202–4.
40. Ibid., p. 206.
41. The novel was *Seiyūki*, or *Xiyouji* in Chinese. It was a grand novel based on traditional stories about a T'ang dynasty monk's travels to India.

Village Officials, Poetry
Circles, Religious and Cultural Activities

Keisaku's book-lending network consisted not only of doctors but also of poets, officials, and other educated members of the local elite. These relationships provide a good picture of the way private circles overlapped with official ones. Nagai Jōzan (Ryūsuke), for example, was another prominent village official from Yokō. As a fellow official, Keisaku shared with Jōzan the official business of the village. On a personal level, too, they had much in common. Like Keisaku, Jōzan was a wealthy farmer who had interests in silk farming. He was a painter and exchanged books with Keisaku on subjects such as *haikai* poetry, Confucianism, and Dutch grammar. Perhaps the most significant indication of the way their public and private interests overlapped is that Keisaku entrusted Jōzan's two sons in marriage to his two daughters, Kano and Kato. Thus related by the marriage of their children, they shared a close and binding relationship.

Keisaku was also close to his brother-in-law Nara Anpei (1809–65), who lived in nearby Ōzuka village and was married to Kono, the younger sister of Keisaku's first wife. Like Keisaku, Anpei was a wealthy farmer and a distinguished local poet. Throughout the diary, Keisaku recounts visiting him on a regular basis, often staying the night. At least one of these visits was a *renga* poetry party hosted by Anpei (1855.2.5). The two loaned each other books of poetry, and it was Anpei whom Keisaku trusted to correct his *waka* poetry. When Kono fell ill, Keisaku treated her intensively, and as noted above, her death appears to have caused a lapse in the diary.

Keisaku's status as a village official gave him many important connections to others of similar standing. Not least of these was his relationship with Negishi Kenbei (Kenroku) of Isemachi, who was employed as the *daikan* (intendant) of the seven villages in the area. Kenbei had duties at the official residence of the *hatamoto* overlord in Edo every second month and was thus an important source of news for those who remained in the village. For example, he passed on news that he received about the activities of the Americans, as noted by Keisaku in the following entry: "It is said that the

Americans have been granted 3,000 *tsubo* of land in Shimoda, in Izu province, to land their ships. The American ship is still in the bay in Izu. Negishi [Kenbei] said that he received a letter from the Hoshina (*hatamoto*) residence in Edo" (1854.4.6). There is evidence that Kenbei purchased and brought back *rangaku* books that Keisaku requested from Edo (1857.2.24). Furthermore, during the 1830s, Kenbei seems to have served as messenger and coordinator of correspondence between Chōei and the group in Kōzuke (1839.9.12). This means that the highest local representative of Bakufu authority in the village was not only "on-side," he was an intimate member of their circle of acquaintance.

Something of the breadth of Keisaku's role as an educator and local intellectual in his community may be seen from his involvement in poetry circles. He was a keen poet and served as a local adjudicator, or *tenja*, for many surrounding villages. He consistently recorded the requests he received for *haikai* adjudications in his diary and sometimes also the remuneration he received for this work. Interestingly, many of these requests were associated with village shrines. In such cases, Keisaku was probably employed to make a selection of outstanding poems that would be framed and presented to the gods at the local shrine. The devotion usually included a prayer for continued progress in writing poetry.[42] As we have seen, he sometimes dedicated his own poems to the local Shinto shrine, too.

Poetry or "elegant" parties were an important part of the social scene. Those Keisaku attended appear to have been intense affairs, often lasting two or three days, and with a period of consultation and anticipation before the event. For a party held by his friend Hokkei of Arigawa village in 1857, he was wooed with *sake* and snacks several days in advance in order to persuade him to write a flyer for the event (1857.7.17). He stayed two nights at the party; the whole day between was spent writing, painting, and drawing (1857.7.29). Two weeks later, the same group of poetry friends (including the poetess Morita Kōgetsu) gathered again for a moon-viewing, and Keisaku stayed another two nights at Hokkei's house

---

42. Aoki Toshiyuki, personal communication, September 1999.

(1857.8.15). If the diary is any indication, such parties were held quite infrequently, and the gatherings themselves appear to have been less important than the relationships they fostered. Hokkei, for example, was a frequent visitor at Keisaku's house. He often came bearing gifts of *sake*, which presumably the two shared. In another example of a poetic gathering, in the following year a group of Keisaku's beginning poetry students brought some wine, and they wrote poetry together until daybreak to commemorate the death of the poet Bashō (1858.10.12).

The poetess Morita Kōgetsu, of Iwamoto village, has already been introduced as the conveyor of the cowpox lymph that Keisaku used to vaccinate his grandchildren. Kōgetsu was the niece of the well-respected poet Gotsū. When her uncle died, she asked Keisaku to write the inscription for his memorial tablet and had him organize a special poetry session in his memory (1855.3.28). Kōgetsu associated with Keisaku over a period of many years (gradually he came to call her "old Kōgetsu"). Eventually, she came to live with a wealthy merchant in Nakanojō (1871.8.22).

Another contact Keisaku made through his interest in poetry was Inō Setsuryō. Setsuryō was a village headman from Iwamoto, where Keisaku had many poetic friends. Although Setsuryō was seventeen years younger than Keisaku, he became a regular visitor after 1860, often bearing gifts of *sake* and staying the night. Together, they seem to have been involved in a *kōshin* religious fraternity, and on more than one occasion, the purpose of Setsuryō's visit was to ask Keisaku to write the inscription for religious stone monuments (for example, 1862.1.18).

There is an interesting relationship between the *kōshin* religion and medicine. Originally, the religion came from a Taoist tradition that there were three worms that lived in the head, stomach, and lower part of the human body. They were present in the human body from birth, and each worm was associated with one of three human desires: for material wealth, food and drink, and sexual gratification. The word *kōshin* referred to a year or day in the Chinese sexagenary cycle. On these nights, it was believed that the worms, who knew all about one's human failings, would creep away in one's sleep to reveal one's sins to the gods and thus shorten one's life. Therefore, people stayed awake on these nights.[43] As the tradition became associated with Buddhism, priests and ascetics, who often served as healers, encouraged the formation of *kōshin* groups all over the country. Yamazaki Ansai called for a "Japanese" *kōshin* religion and associated it with the Japanese god Sarudahiko no Mikoto. Thus, the religion had Buddhist, Shinto, and ascetic versions, and the wakeful night ranged from a time for reflection to an all-night party.[44]

The worms themselves were sometimes conceived of as godly and sometimes as ordinary parasitic worms. The religious and medical aspects of the tradition became confused, and the three worms were often associated with common medical problems such as colic. Indeed, the story of the worms was included in Japan's oldest medical book, the *Ishinpō*. Even when the role of healing began to be filled by secular doctors rather than Buddhist priests, *kōshin* ideas continued to be propagated by medical men.[45] Perhaps Keisaku's strong association with the *kōshin* religious fraternity reflects this traditional relationship.

Keisaku's poetic skills and interest in Western studies seem to have served him well when he visited Edo on official business in 1857. At the time, he was employed as the village headman and made the customary New Year's trip to the residence of the *hatamoto* overseer of the village, Tominaga Magorokurō. Tominaga appears to have been interested in Western learning, for during Keisaku's visit he asked to see an original Dutch book, which Keisaku gave to him, and Keisaku in turn was ordered to go and inspect a collection of Dutch grammar books at the house of Tominaga's relative. Upon Tominaga's request, Keisaku gave him two notebooks of poems he had written and requested poetry notebooks in return from Tominaga and his wife (1.14, 1.16). This kind of exchange demonstrates something of the privileged position village officials such as Keisaku held when it came to obtaining

---

43. Shirasugi, "Senki to Edo jidai no hitobito no shintai keiken," pp. 80–83.
44. See Kokushi Daijiten Henshū Iinkai, ed., *Kokushi daijiten*, 5: 397–99.
45. Shirasugi, "Senki to Edo jidai no hitobito no shintai keiken," pp. 80–83.

information and the way in which literary pursuits such as poetry facilitated social and professional interaction.

This trip was quite an adventure for Keisaku, for it is the only one he made to Edo throughout the entire period of the diary. Reading the diary, it is possible to imagine that he never wanted to go again thereafter. Despite the fact that he rode a horse for much of the journey, he complained of a sore knee and muscle pain that was "extremely hard to bear" (1857.1.9). After he returned, he suffered from infected blisters on his toes, which gave him a burning pain that made walking difficult and forced him to send his son Keisuke to attend to his duties in his place (1.25). The pain did not even begin to ease until twelve days after his return, and he does not appear to have gone anywhere for about a month.

Not only was Keisaku a respected poet, he was also a calligrapher and was interested in art. He kept a sizable collection of paintings, scrolls, and decorated fans. The diary records innumerable instances in which his artwork was commissioned by friends and neighbors. Sometimes he made a note at the end of the year of the money he received for his paintings, writing, and poems (1860.12.30). It does not appear to have been a large sum (a little over one *ryō* for 1860), but the fact that he recorded it suggests that it had a certain significance for him. As a further example of Keisaku's role as an authority in his community, in 1869, when people were required to change their personal names to fit certain specifications, villagers came to him for help in choosing their new names (1869.10.1, 1869.12.28, 1871.3.11).

Travelers

Poetry, medical, and social circles came into play when traveling poets, artists, and scholars were passing through town. Travelers often came with letters of introduction supplied by members of a network. From the diary, it can be seen that Keisaku played host to many poets and scholars from faraway places. These visitors included priests from Mt. Haruna and Shinshū and doctors from Shikanuma (now Tochigi prefecture), Echigo (Niigata), Osaka (though Keisaku was absent and missed him), Kanazawa (Ishikawa), and Kyoto. Traveling poets and calligraphers visited from places such

such as Echigo, Numata, and Edo. Depending on how well he liked the visitors, Keisaku might give them money or board for a night. For example, in 1865 he wrote, "A medical student by the name of Satō Jun'an visited from the post-station of Kōnosu. He was quite a calligrapher; so I gave him one *shu* in coins" (1865.5.26).

In 1863, a Chōshū Confucian scholar by the name of Sekiguchi came bearing a letter of introduction from Gakkai, a priestly associate of Keisaku who was interested in poetry and painting. At the time, his house was in a mess and he felt unable to put up the visiting scholar, but he took him instead to the house of his chief medical student, Gōsai. Keisaku also wrote the visitor an introduction to a house in Nakanojō (1863.6.6). In this way, travelers could literally move along a chain of social networks forged by common interest.

Wealthy rural commoners such as Keisaku were usually happy to have new company and stimulation. When he had a visit from a poet by the name of Gen'a in 1864, he enthused that their discussions about poetry were "extremely interesting." Gen'a stayed five nights before Keisaku sent him on to Isemachi with an introduction to Kenbei (1864.8.23).

Sometime in the 1830s, Takano Chōei wrote a letter to Teizō introducing his friend Fukuda Hanka, visiting from Edo:

The bearer of this letter is called Fukuda Hanka, one of the closest of my friends. He is a landscape painter, and since he was keen to visit the area, he asked me to write a letter of introduction to [you and to] Sawatari too. His character is certainly not that of an aimless wanderer: he is a very upright and warm-hearted man. Please look after him. He would like to earn a little money; so I hope you will help him in this respect too. Please talk to Keisaku and be so kind as to act as his guide. Fukuda will tell you all about my circumstances. I will write everything in a later letter. In the meantime, I write in haste to ask you this favor. Please give my best regards to your wife.

> 16th day of the New Year
> Takano Chōei
> To Yanagida Teizō-*sama*[46]

Travelers were great sources of information. As Tessa Morris-Suzuki has noted in her *Technological Transformation of Japan*, the

---

46. Takano Chōun, *Takano Chōei den*, p. 316.

benefits of travel for the spread of technology were well recognized by domains, which "encouraged a small but significant direct flow of skilled workers from one district to another."[47] As can be seen from Keisaku's diary, private travel also had an important role to play in bringing news and knowledge. For example, when a pharmacist from Shinshū visited Keisaku a few days after the great Kanto Earthquake in 1853, he brought news of damage done in the provinces of Kai and Izu (1853.11.18). When a doctor from Kanazawa came, he stayed two nights and Keisaku talked about medical matters with him "all day." He recorded in the same entry the titles of several medical books, presumably recommended by the visitor (1861.3.8).

Often, members of the rural elite seem to have shared their special visitors with others in their circle. For example, when the Numata calligrapher Ubukata Teisai (1795–1856) visited Teizō in 1839, Keisaku went along to meet him, participated in a sightseeing day trip to Sawatari, and stayed the night at Teizō's house (1839.4.25). From Takano Chōei's letter above, it can be imagined that a similar expedition was arranged for Fukuda Hanka.

Keisaku often appears to have met other doctors at the local pharmacies, which were natural gathering places for those interested in medicine. Drinking establishments were another source of interesting contacts. At Negishi Shūzō's business, which was both pharmacy and brewery, the two naturally overlapped. One of the more unusual examples of Keisaku's visitors was a retired sumo wrestler from Edo, whom he met at one of his regular drinking places when he called in on his way home from a fishing expedition. He gave the visitor some fish, and as he was apparently interested in elegant pursuits, he invited him home to stay the night (1863.9.22).

Old Age

As he became older, Keisaku's students became an increasingly important part of his life. They came to him at various stages of their lives and for various reasons. Many of the youngest students

---

47. Morris-Suzuki, *The Technological Transformation*, p. 33.

were the children of local village officials who came to polish their literacy skills. Others came to read the Confucian classics or to study poetry, calligraphy, *rangaku*, and medicine. The older students became friends, drinking partners, and colleagues with whom to share information and books. Although Keisaku recorded the instances when students first came to him, he unfortunately did not usually give details of the lessons thereafter. Poetry students often appear to have come in groups, whereas other promising students were given individual attention. The frequency of lessons also appears to have varied. The eight-year-old son of Keisaku's closest disciple came for lessons four or five times a month, whereas older students visited much less often, presumably because they had other commitments. Keisaku appears to have written many "model texts" that he gave to students to study and copy. Upon request he would give lectures on specific books, such as certain of the Confucian classics or medical books (1860.10.12, 1868.3.7).

Far from spending a quiet retirement, Keisaku was encouraged by his students to remain academically active right up until he died. In 1874, the final year of the diary, Keisaku spent the entire year working on an anatomical book called *Zentai shinron* (New thesis on the whole body). Koitabashi Ryōsaburō, successor to the Koitabashi pharmacy, brought the book to Keisaku early in the year, requesting that they read it together (1874.1.25). It was not long before another medical student joined in. Not only did Keisaku read it with his students, he was inspired to write a commentary on it, which he spent the remainder of the year writing and revising. *Zentai shinron* was written in Chinese by the English medical missionary Benjamin Hobson (1816–73). It was published in Shanghai in 1851 but was not printed in Japan until 1857. Although he probably did not know it, Keisaku was actually beaten to the post by Ishiguro Atsushi, who translated and published the work as *Zentai shinron yakkai* that same year.[48]

---

48. Nichiran Gakkai, ed., *Yōgakushi jiten*, p. 401.

Eighteen seventy-four was also the year in which Yokō village opened its own school, in the hall of the village temple.[49] Keisaku made a generous donation of fifteen yen to the school and attended all day for the first two days of classes. In consultation with the local administrator, who was a longtime student and friend, he researched and wrote the school regulations. He was also in close contact with one of the first teachers there, Seki Saburō. The two exchanged books and read school texts, such as Fukuzawa Yukichi's *Gakumon no susume*, together (1874.9.15, 12.9).

In the early Meiji period, Keisaku's life as a doctor and local intellectual continued much as it always had. As long as official policy did not begin to encroach too much on the rhythms of his daily life, he appears to have been content not to comment on events in the wider political realm, at least in his diary. He was the kind of man who, when there was a ban on the traditional celebration of "little new year" in 1867 due to the recent death of the Emperor Kōmei, simply made his rice cakes secretly at night.[50] Perhaps his failure to acquiesce reflects where his true loyalties lay.

It is clear that Keisaku was not always happy with the changes that he saw around him. In 1868, in the midst of a spate of looting and arson attempts on the houses of local well-to-dos, he complained: "the lawlessness of the world is truly frightening" (1868.3.28). Again, he was quite critical of the new government's policies: "The national laws are still undecided. The official notices are all sent out in the morning, only to be revised in the evening. Many of the taxes on transportation and the like are unfair. In the first notice about silk farming, we were asked to write down the yield for the last five years, now it is thirteen!" (1872.3.29).

---

49. After the beginning of the Meiji period, the influence of Shinto in the village was extremely strong. Perhaps the Buddhist temple was all but unused. See Kanai, *Takahashi Keisaku nikki*, p. 513.

50. Emperor Kōmei died in the twelfth month of 1866. *Koshōgatsu* was celebrated around the fifteenth of the first month according to the lunar calendar and, along with the making of rice cakes, involved several kinds of festivities related to agriculture.

Despite his interest in Western medicine, Keisaku appears to have been wary of the Westernization of Japanese culture. In 1867, he wrote:

According to the orders of the shogunate, the various military families gradually have begun to wear foreign-style clothing, let their hair and beards grow long, and have ruffles at the wrist. Clothing is sewn together and of foreign origin, people wear shoes when they present themselves at the castle, and sit on chairs even in front of their superiors. Japanese customs are disappearing more and more, and to see the way they are assimilated into Western ones is vexing and truly a terrible shame.   (1867.2.30)

Keisaku made a note in his diary of new pharmaceutical standards in 1874 (8.31), but did not mention the laws passed in the same month that made examinations in Western medicine compulsory for all new practicing physicians. It was Keisaku's students, rather than he, who had to deal with these changes. One wonders whether Keisaku would have taken these changes in his stride, much in the same way as he embraced the new school system, had he lived. His students certainly kept him up to date with the latest developments. In the year before he died, in addition to working on his commentary for *Zentai shinron*, he copied a clipping of a Tokyo newspaper with news that Gotō Shōbun had developed a treatment for leprosy (1874.4.14). In the same year he was reading Japan's first medical journal, Tsuboi Shinryō's *Iji zasshi* (1874.6.22). This journal was published by Shinryō in monthly installments in the years 1873–75. It contained translations and annotations of new theories discussed in Dutch medical circles.[51]

Ranpō Medicine and Modernity

Nevertheless, there is some evidence that the changes occurring in the field of medicine during the Meiji period were not always easy to cope with, even for students who had been trained to an extent in *rangaku*. Seki Gōsai (1844–1907) was Keisaku's closest disciple. The first mention of him made in the diary was in 1857, when Keisaku sent him to the pharmacy in Isemachi on an errand (5.12). Al-

---

51. Nichiran Gakkai, ed., *Yōgakushi jiten*, p. 122.

though it is unclear whether he actually lived with Keisaku, he appears to have been an apprentice in a true sense, for he was also required to help out with silk reeling, weeding, and other household tasks (1857.inter 5.18, 6.7). By the time of the epidemic in 1862, Gōsai was making visits as a locum for his teacher. Keisaku gave him the freedom to set up an independent practice in 1863, at the age of nineteen (1863.4.3). Nevertheless, the two continued to maintain a firm friendship, and Keisaku began teaching Gōsai's son, Gōzō (who later became a dentist), in 1871 (3.5).

On the other hand, Gōsai had also been studying *kokugaku* with the Shinto priest Koitabashi Yoshisato and became devoted to the imperial cause.[52] In 1873, he was appointed to the local Shinto shrine. In 1877, after Keisaku's death, he gave up this post and made a return to medicine, entering the prefectural medical school. He passed the medical examinations in 1879 and gained an appointment at a public hospital. Shortly before he was meant to take up his post and begin private practice in Numata, however, he suddenly had a change of heart and decided instead to go to Tokyo. His objective was to study *rangaku* and surgery and become a military doctor. Before departing, he visited Fukuda Bundō (Sōtei's son) in Sawatari to ask for a letter of introduction to the army doctor Hayashi Kenkai (1844–82), son of the leading *rangaku* scholar Hayashi Dōkai (1813–95).[53] But when he met Dōkai in Tokyo, he was told that *rangaku*'s heyday was already over and that he should learn French or German instead. Furthermore, at the age of 36, he was already too old to become a military doctor. For lessons in surgery, he should approach Satō Taizen of the Juntendō school. Gōsai, however, remained adamant. He wanted to learn *rangaku*. He could still remember some of what he had learned when young, and at his age, surely it would be better to continue with Dutch

---

52. The information in this section is based on selections from Gōsai's *Tokyo Diary*, introduced in Kanai, "Rangaku to waga Nakanojōmachi," pp. 1146–51; and Kanai, *Takano Chōei to Agatsuma*, pp. 38–39.

53. Fukuda Bundō (1841–87) had studied under Hayashi Dōkai in Edo, but the letter of introduction was to his son, Kenkai. Perhaps this was because Gōsai expressed an interest in a military medical career. In Tokyo, Gōsai appears to have met Kenkai first and then requested a meeting with his father.

than begin a new language. But no matter how he pleaded, Dōkai would not agree, and Gōsai, who had run out of money, turned dejectedly homeward, selling his books and clothing to pay for his journey. He returned to private medical practice and to the Shinto faith, opening a private school, which he called Kōdōgakkan (Hall of learning for the imperial way).

Actually, Gōsai's desire to study more *rangaku* may not have been his own, but his teacher Keisaku's. In a letter to Fukuda Bundō, Gōsai wrote, "I cannot throw away the instructions given me by my deceased teacher. Even if this field of learning continues to decline and one day becomes obsolete, I will have not the slightest regret about becoming outdated with it."[54] Gōsai was already a qualified medical practitioner, and he had no practical need to study *rangaku* texts any further. Indeed, the study of *rangaku*, and the Dutch language in particular, had become something quite divorced from the study of modern Western medicine, at least in official terms. In 1870, the Japanese government decided that Western medicine would be introduced on the basis of a German model, and a succession of German professors was invited to teach in Japan. The study of the Dutch language and the translation of Dutch texts became practically obsolete. Gōsai's journey to Tokyo is best seen as a tribute to his teacher Keisaku, who had left him with the legacy of a dying art. It was Gōsai, rather than Keisaku, who had the uncomfortable experience of trying to straddle two worlds and discovering that the one he knew best had lost its meaning.

Similarly, it was the new generation of local doctors who began to experience the professionalization of medicine. They undertook formal schooling and examinations, were appointed to newly established hospitals, and joined professional medical associations. It was a world far removed from that in which local doctors, with little sense of territorial competition, studied together and shared books and knowledge and even patients.

Some scholars have discussed the importance of *rangaku* in terms of the creation of a social foundation for modernization. Bartholomew, for example, noted the importance of Western stud-

---

54. Kanai, "Rangaku to waga Nakanojōmachi," p. 1149.

ies in the Tokugawa period, not for intellectual development but for recruiting talented scholars to science after 1868.[55] Goodman granted *rangaku* a role in fostering a "curiosity about the West" and helping scholars to identify European techniques as superior, which assisted in smoothing the way for the rapid assimilation of Western knowledge in the Meiji period.[56]

One must be wary of interpreting the changeover from *rangaku* to Western medicine that was led by these men as a simple or linear process. Seki Gōsai retrained and served his community as a doctor of Western medicine in the early Meiji period. In this sense, he may be seen as one of *rangaku*'s recruits to modern medicine. However, the story of his aborted trip to Edo to study surgery and *rangaku* demonstrates that his belief in the value of *rangaku* was not to be equated with a belief in the path to the new, Western modernity. Gōsai studied Western medicine as was required of him by new laws, but this did not prevent him from wanting to study Dutch, despite the fact that he knew it was outdated. Here we see the gap that historian Numata Jirō perceived between *rangaku* and modern Western science[57] and can perceive that "progress" did not always occur in the patterns we might expect.

Nevertheless, it is important to remember that nineteenth-century European medical practice was yet to enter the age of bacteriological discovery. Physicians in Europe and America as well as in Japan were struggling to come to terms with the implications that science held for medicine. During the long Tokugawa period, a slow process of medical change took place, brought about in response to the assimilation of both Chinese and Western medicine in Japan and their subsequent development. By the time the Meiji government passed the law requiring all physicians to study Western medicine, the Japanese physicians were in a similar position to their Western counterparts, who, together with a new generation of Japanese scholars, were to undertake enormous theoretical steps early in the twentieth century. That Japanese scientists such as

---

55. Bartholomew, *The Formation of Science in Japan*, p. 4.
56. Goodman, *Japan: The Dutch Experience*, p. 234.
57. See pp. 15–16.

Kitazato Shibasaburō (1852–1931) played an important role in such research is a sure indication of this.

Gōnō, Literacy, and Networks

An examination of Keisaku's diary reveals that it is impossible to consider his work as a country medical practitioner separately from his position in the community as a farmer, village official, poet, and calligrapher. Apart from the time when the village was struck by an epidemic, his medical practice was never a full-time occupation. Perhaps he is best thought of as a rural intellectual who liked to participate in the various fields of learning that his education had made available to him and who developed a wide range of skills that enabled him to participate effectively in many of them. These interests were shared with other members of the rural elite, some of whom were relatives, other doctors, or well-to-do farmers. He may be said to typify the new class of educated rural entrepreneur or gōnō that is commonly credited with an important role in Japan's economic and political modernization.

When characterizing Dutch studies in Japan, Grant Goodman wrote in 1986 that "rangaku was never a 'grassroots' movement and did not reflect any demands from below."[58] If Goodman's statement is considered against the evidence in this book, perhaps it is true to the extent that doctors such as the Kōzuke physicians, as members of a local elite, were of an "in-between" status, by no means at the lowest level of society. Yet at the same time they were operating on a level quite different from official domain or Bakufu doctors.

The men behind medicine's move into the countryside were in many cases gōnō. Their wealth and high level of education (often undertaken in the cities) supplied them with the financial and intellectual means and necessary leisure to pursue the study of medicine, while business and official connections provided them with information and an abundance of patients. As discussed in Chapter 1, a

---

58. Goodman, *Japan: The Dutch Experience*, p. 7.

link may be seen between village officials' privileged access to medical information and their propensity to become doctors.

Village officials had a role in the dissemination of both information and medicines. Such displays of benevolence were meant to reinforce the Tokugawa political system. In the area of public health, for example, Takahashi Keisaku recorded in his diary an official notice that recommended certain treatments for cholera. Brett Walker has discussed the role of sponsored smallpox vaccinations of the Ainu population in Hokkaido as a part of the Tokugawa Bakufu's attempts to bring these people into its political realm.[59]

Central to the elite villagers' access to official information was their literacy. As discussed by Tsukamoto Manabu in extensive writings about the relationship between literacy, medicine, and authority, the rise of literacy in the countryside during the Edo period was brought about initially through a need for written communication between the samurai class in the cities and the village officials who administered in their absence.[60] It was in the interest of village officials not only to be able to read and write but to know the correct expressions to make legal and other applications. Style books were popular, and the trends of the warrior class were copied by villagers in their writing.[61]

Tsukamoto has argued that there was a gap between members of the ruling class, who learned their writing from Chinese culture, and commoners, who learned from city culture as it spread. City learning tended to be based on classical studies, whereas village learning was practical and concrete. For village officials, written culture could be perceived as a way to gain recognition of their rights by the ruling class.[62]

Anne Walthall has argued in a similar vein that many rural elites began to keep family records, such as diaries, in order to "define a place for themselves and their families." As they gained new power and wealth in their communities, they needed to legitimize their

---

59. Walker, "The Early Modern Japanese State and Ainu Vaccinations: Redefining the Body Politic, 1799–1868."
60. Tsukamoto, *Tokai to inaka*, p. 193.
61. Tsukamoto, "Toshi bunka to no kōryū," pp. 356–59.
62. Ibid., pp. 364, 376.

position by creating a family tradition.[63] Literacy was therefore a powerful tool by which elites could distinguish themselves from ordinary commoners.

Tsukamoto's "gap," however, must be viewed with a certain degree of suspicion, at least when considering the better-educated village officials. Moriya has suggested that there was "no great difference, in terms of literacy, between peasant officialdom and samurai."[64] Although villagers may have had interests different from those of urban samurai, their down-to-earth "practicality" did not prevent them from writing poetry in both Chinese and Japanese (as did Fukuda Sōtei and Takahashi Keisaku) or abstract Confucian essays (as did Keisaku's teacher in Shinano, Itō Chūtai). Some, like Fukuda Sōtei, spent long years studying in prestigious private academies in the cities and were therefore as well educated as many samurai.

As might be expected, there was some variation in the level of literary skill achieved by village officials. In a diary entry for 1868, Keisaku recorded that, in recent years, the use of Chinese expressions in official documents had increased, making them difficult for village officials to read. People were beginning to come from here and there to ask his help in reading them. He roundly criticized the impertinence and lack of consideration of the rulers in circulating such documents (1868.1.16).

There are interesting parallels between the spread of written culture and the acceptance of medicine into villages. Tsukamoto has suggested that the flow of medicine from towns to villages rode on the wave of a new dependency on the written word. In the absence of a system of registration, it was easy for anyone who had read a few medical books to set himself up as a doctor. With the arrival of accessible medical treatment in the countryside in the form of these *gōnō* doctors, villagers gradually began to replace their traditional folklore based on an oral tradition with faith in a medicine based on written culture.[65] Slowly, the idea began to take root that when one

---

63. Walthall, "The Family Ideology of the Rural Entrepreneurs," pp. 464–66.
64. Moriya, "Urban Networks and Information Networks," p. 118.
65. Tsukamoto, *Tokai to inaka*, p. 212.

became sick, the natural thing to do was to seek the advice of a doctor. As a consequence, ordinary villagers became more dependent on local doctors, who were already members of the rural elite and in many cases in a position of authority through their roles as village officials. It was a growing dependence on formal medical knowledge, of course, that would eventually facilitate the success of state-sponsored medicine in the late Tokugawa period and beyond.

Well-educated rural physicians were in a unique position because they had access to both written Chinese knowledge and more traditional, orally transmitted, local knowledge. Perhaps this was a factor in the success of the cooperation between Takano Chōei and his farmer-physician friends in Kōzuke, when they wrote about crops and famine relief in 1836. Equipped with both hands-on practical experience and the authority of the written word, rural physicians were in an ideal position to gain the trust of their local communities.

Far from being simply the ability to read official notices and write tax reports, literacy was to many rural elites the very axis of their social worlds. As may be seen from the social life of Takahashi Keisaku, literacy gave rural physicians a powerful tool not only for their working lives but also for leisure. Many rural elites devoted their spare time to aesthetic pursuits such as poetry, calligraphy, and study. Due to their popularity and the way in which they were enjoyed, aesthetic pursuits were by no means lonely or isolating, even in rural areas. Just as city scholars and literary figures gathered to socialize and share ideas and activities, rural elites held their own poetry parties, flower-viewings, and study meetings.

Tanaka Yūko has shown how *haikai* poetry networks all over the country could be used as a highly effective distribution system. In 1762, Western enthusiast Hiraga Gennai (1728–79) was the organizer of an enormously successful exhibition in Edo of 1,300 botanical specimens from all over the country. According to Tanaka, he owed his success to a series of collection points he set up in many regions, so that people might bring in their specimens. These collection points were pre-existing, used by *haikai* poetry networks.[66]

---

66. Tanaka, *Edo no sōzōryoku*, p. 66.

Thus, as may be seen from the life of Takahashi Keisaku in rural Kōzuke, *gōnō* farmers were in an ideal position to experiment with medicine, just as they did with sericulture and other technologies. Far from living an isolated existence, members of the rural elite in nineteenth-century rural Japan were connected by many different "synapses." The social networks of the rural *gōnō* contained a dynamic mixture of overlapping medical, literary, commercial, and official circles. These networks facilitated the flow of information, including that concerning *rangaku*, into rural Japan, and fostered an interest in practical pursuits, social welfare, and social change.

CONCLUSION
Ranpō *Medicine and*
Practical Pursuits

Ranpō doctors in Tokugawa Japan did not generally understand European medical knowledge in the scientific terms in which it was later formally introduced. Yet this is not to say that their efforts had no meaning. This book has discussed the dynamic ways in which Western medicine spread through social networks and brought doctors together in practical efforts at social change. The haphazard adoption of Western knowledge in this period was not simply a failure to absorb an immutable body of scientific knowledge but a creative and adaptive exercise with a practical end. This approach presents an alternative to the narrative of "Westernization" put forward in some previous histories of *rangaku*.

Throughout the book, the primary concern has been the Japanese interpretation of Western knowledge, rather than its European roots. What was *done* with the knowledge obtained through *rangaku* scholarship has been the point, rather than *rangaku*'s relation to European medical science. The specific case studies involving Takano Chōei and Takahashi Keisaku have provided a detailed picture of the context into which Western knowledge was introduced and the geographical spaces and social networks that supported uses of that knowledge. Through an examination of *ranpō* medicine's practical applications and its social impact at the level of everyday life, it is possible to see it as something far more meaningful and creative than the muddled absorption of supposed facts, which were often inaccurate.

Taking a social rather than a political approach to the history of *rangaku* has also enabled a re-examination of the history of Takano Chōei, one of its central figures. There was far more to Chōei's scholarship than his famous criticism of the "shell and repel" edict in *The Tale of a Dream* in 1838. He himself appears to have found it difficult to reconcile himself to the idea that a paper so divorced from his true interests caused him so much strife. His early reputation was built on his medical scholarship, and the lectures and works on famine relief and epidemic disease discussed in this book help to present an image of Chōei as a socially conscious man of medicine, rather than as a political activist.

A social approach to the history of Western medicine in Japan also helps to provide an alternative to a straightforward narrative of "progress" and the history of discovery. We have seen instead how medical practitioners lived, trained, and worked in the Edo period, how they identified themselves as members of various intellectual groups, and how they struggled to find places for themselves within the social hierarchy.

One of the aims of this study has been to explore the introduction of Western medicine in places other than the large cities or the schools of famous scholars. By the late nineteenth century, Western medical knowledge, in the form of *ranpō* medicine, had permeated the countryside all over Japan. This knowledge, brought to communities by local physicians, touched the lives of ordinary people in the areas that mattered most: health, sustenance, and the education of their children.

The increasing influence of commercial medicine in rural areas of Japan, particularly from the nineteenth century on, developed against a background of social and economic change. Improved communications and increased travel and tourism in the latter part of the Edo period assisted the spread of information and culture, as well as the circulation of commodities such as drugs, including Western ones. Cheap, commercial medical preparations came to be peddled all over the countryside, further increasing the interest of the general populace in medicine. Improvements in communications naturally also facilitated scholarly and cultural exchanges, supported by particular community networks. As demonstrated in

Chapter 3, Nakanojō village in Kōzuke, with mountain herbs and thermal springs close at hand, as well as good access to drugs and commodities through its role as a market town and post station, was a particularly suitable venue for medical practice and exchange.

In 1833, Chōei presented a lecture series in Nakanojō based on material from his recently published book on Western medicine. Not only were the country physicians there interested enough to come along and listen to highly specialized and innovative theoretical lectures on Western medicine, but the notes Takahashi Keisaku took at the lectures have a history of their own. They were later copied by his teacher, Itō Chūtai, in Shinano. Since Chūtai, in turn, had an extensive book-lending network, the ripples made by Chōei's visit continued to undulate long after his departure. This gives an important example of the speed with which new ideas could be spread. Chōei's visit of 1833 was followed by many exchanges with the Kōzuke physicians by letter and finally, in 1836, by the two collaborative works, *Treatise on Two Things for the Relief of Famine* and *Methods of Avoiding Epidemic Diseases.*

These two documents provide an example of the way in which Western knowledge was adapted to the Japanese local context. It is helpful to regard this process in terms of the traditional concept of *jitsugaku* (practical learning). Scholars such as Chōei selected, translated, and interpreted from Dutch source material in the way that was most practically useful to the social community for whom they wrote. In these particular examples, they used knowledge of Western crops and treatments of disease to devise solutions to local problems of hunger and epidemics. In other words, they adapted European knowledge to the Japanese context, and used it in conjunction with what they already knew. There was a remarkable similarity in certain concepts of the body and therapeutics in both Chinese and Western medicine at the time Chōei was writing—an example of this is the notion of "bad air" as a disease factor in both traditions. This similarity surely facilitated the way Chōei assimilated and creatively transformed the new knowledge into something that was meaningful to his readers. Furthermore, an examination of the drugs he and Keisaku used shows the hybrid nature of their medical treatments. In his practice, for example, Keisaku mixed Chinese and Western medicines, sometimes even in the same prescription.

In contrast to ideas that *rangaku* was never a grass-roots movement, the reception and domestication of important elements of *rangaku* in the countryside came about largely through the efforts of wealthy commoner (*gōnō*) doctors such as Keisaku in Kōzuke. Many of these doctors trained in the cities and returned to their villages to engage in medical practice and impart their knowledge to others in the locality. Doctors were in demand not only for their healing skills but also for their ability to teach others. As described in Chapter 2, some villages made special efforts, through supplying subsidized housing, for example, to attract ordinary doctors to their communities to treat their ailments and teach their children. This reflects the growing awareness among commoners, even in rural areas, of the value of literacy. In Kōzuke, Keisaku took students of poetry, calligraphy, and medicine in addition to teaching basic literacy skills. His most prominent medical student, Seki Gōsai, went on to play a leading role as a doctor in the local community.

The kinds of changes going on in nineteenth-century rural Japanese society are reflected in Keisaku's diary, which provides a fascinating glimpse of the daily life of a country doctor in the late Edo period. For Keisaku, at least, and presumably for other village doctors with multiple roles, medicine was not a full-time occupation. Keisaku was also a farmer, poet, local official, and intellectual. Although he did receive some remuneration for his medical activities, farming was nevertheless the basis of his livelihood. Because there was no system of licensing, he competed in an open medical market with other doctors, ranging from highly trained men like himself to religious healers and quacks. Despite the competition, however, he was discriminating about his patients and when he chose to make calls. He was in a position to refuse or reschedule his visits to suit his own convenience.

Unlike their contemporaries in Europe, Japanese local doctors appear to have maintained good relations with one another, without any significant territorial animosity. For example, Keisaku gave his blessing to his apprentice Gōsai when he set up an independent practice in the very next village, without any apparent fear that it would encroach on his own work. Perhaps this was because he was not reliant on medical practice as his only source of income. Such a sense of camaraderie naturally assisted the exchange of knowledge and helped to break down the traditional barriers of secrecy between different schools of medicine. In addition to sharing some patients, local doctors met and exchanged books socially. Study groups such as the one that supported Chōei's visit to Naka-nojō appear to have been a significant influence in creating a local interest in Western learning. This influence manifested itself in activities such as the translation of Dutch books and the cultivation of medicinal plants.

These men, in their various roles as doctors, officials, and village intellectuals, enjoyed important positions in the community as upholders of cultural life. Central to their role was the ability to read and write. In addition to his work as a doctor and village official, for example, Keisaku corrected poems, produced calligraphic artwork, copied books, made personal seals, and wrote monument inscriptions for other villagers. In the early Meiji period, he was actively involved in setting up the first village school. Many parallels may be drawn between Keisaku's community services and attempts by provincial doctors in England to appeal to the community for their status. Keisaku's standing in the local community helped to make him popular as a doctor, and his medical and intellectual successes no doubt expanded his authority. He seems to typify a new kind of country doctor that emerged from the level of the local elite toward the end of the Edo period.

Perhaps it was because they already fulfilled a role as protectors of the community that rural doctors also saw it as part of their work to oversee public health. As members of the rural elite, the relationships they made through their official work provided them with superior information networks. Indeed, the spread of doctors into the countryside helped to create an increasing dependence among ordinary people on written medical knowledge rather than traditional medical practices. Health campaigns, publications such as *Treatise on Two Things for the Relief of Famine* and *Methods of Avoiding Epidemic Diseases*, and vaccination combined well with the pre-existing responsibilities of village officials and members of the local elite. In addition to the philanthropic aims of these activities, they no doubt contributed to the status of their authors and of *rangaku* scholarship as a whole.

The success of Western methods of smallpox vaccination was a very important factor in gaining recognition for *ranpō* medicine from the mid-nineteenth century. In many cases, vaccinations were introduced on the initiative of local *ranpō* doctors. Keisaku, for example, appears to have played a role in obtaining vaccine and immunizing his local community against smallpox. This is another example of the way *ranpō* medicine was beginning to be accepted by even the most ordinary of people and was changing their lives.

So against the background of improved transport and communications, economic development, and a rising class of rural entrepreneurs, *rangaku* and *ranpō* medicine were actively studied and promoted in rural Japan through a system of social networks that were supported by specific geographical locales. By adapting the knowledge obtained through Western scholarship to the local context and the perceived practical needs of ordinary communities, physicians such as Chōei and Keisaku did much to assist the domestication of Western medicine in rural Japan. As new forms of medicine began to permeate the countryside, physicians appear to have played an increasingly important role in their communities as intellectuals, educators, and protectors of public health.

Thus the pursuit of knowledge about Western medicine in Tokugawa Japan was a socially dynamic, intensely practical activity. Despite attempts by the Bakufu to control the importation of this knowledge and the way in which it was used, scholars went to great lengths to obtain it. Far from being monopolized by government and domain officials, Western medical books were being obtained, read, translated, and shared by local doctors all over the countryside. They hungered for such information not only for their own personal satisfaction and the status-enhancing opportunities it might provide, but because they saw that it had practical social applications, in both medicine and social welfare. The study of Western knowledge therefore became a vehicle for the exchange of ideas between urban and rural intellectuals, and, eventually, for social change in the late Tokugawa period and beyond.

Appendixes

Treatise on Two Things for the Relief of Famine

Epigraph

Perhaps there is no greater disaster for the people than a year of poor harvest. Yet the reasons given for crop failure rarely go beyond the two of drought or flood. Our country's soil and paddies are fertile and crossed in all directions by rivers and marshes; so the people do not often suffer from drought. However, problems of flooding are extremely severe. It is of great concern that in recent years this has been occurring frequently.[1]

In all probability, the people of our country take their sustenance exclusively from rice, wheat, and barley. However, it takes a long time for these crops to mature. And in addition, in the temperate zones at the time of the equinox, there are frequent violent storms, which uproot trees and blow down roofs. In such cases, the damage is not only to paddies and soil but directly to the people. If such storms should occur at a time when it has been damp and cold for months, and the rice, barley, and wheat have not matured, what could one do to avoid starvation?

Ah, how the farmers give their energies to farming! Although showered with rain and combed by the wind, irritated by sweat

---

1. For further discussion of this document, see Chapter 4, pp. 118–24.

and the oil on their skins all dried up, they work untiringly and look forward to the harvest, only to meet with such disaster and have their efforts evaporate all at once. How can one not feel sorry for them? Accordingly, such a great calamity is not just that of the farmers, but of society at large. Even though these are prosperous times now and there are few who starve to death, if the price of rice jumps, then a day's work is not enough to buy a day's food. With regard to this matter, in desolate villages and cold hamlets, it comes to scraping the bark from trees or washing the muddy earth to eat. By doing so, people are able to ward off starvation for a time, but because such foods are unusual, within one or two, or perhaps three or four months, there are many who fall ill and die. This is the reason why there is much sickness after a poor harvest. I am always worried by this.

Consider this. Although the countries near the North Pole are intensely, bitingly cold, and there are only one or two months a year in which the ice melts, why do the people there not starve? It is because they plant things to eat that do not fear wind, cold, heat, or damp. I have always thought it a pity that we did not have the seeds of those plants. This year [1836] the rain and damp has continued from the third month to the eighth month, with very few fine days in between. It is colder than 1833. In each province there has been flooding, the price of rice has gradually become more expensive, and people, in their concern, cannot still their beating hearts.

In the middle of the eighth month of this year, I met Fukuda Sōtei of Sawatari in Jōmō [Kōzuke]. The Sōteis have for generations been surgeons by profession and are very skilled in their art. Also, Sōtei reads Dutch books in order to study the subject further. I have enjoyed a warm relationship with him from the beginning, and one evening, just when our conversation was getting in full swing, he pulled out a scoop of buckwheat and showed it to me, saying, "In general, the reason why people die in a bad year is because they do not have enough to eat. And the reason why there is not enough food is because there are not any crops that can be harvested several times a year. This buckwheat should mature three times a year. Do you not think that it would be a great treasure for the poor people?"

I was very surprised and grateful, and replied, "When people in the countries near the North Pole choose their crops, they choose ones that grow quickly. If these crops were grown in a warm area, they would mature several times a year. The reason why I have wanted these plants was to grow them here and increase the yield and prevent starvation. In the past I have looked for them in faraway places and suddenly now I find them so near! Although given to me by you, in truth it is a gift from heaven!"

I took [the buckwheat] gladly. Later I was given a type of tuber by a man called Yanagida Teizō, from Isemachi in the same province. Upon examination, it was shaped like a yam and also like a *hodoimo*.[2] According to local custom it is called a Jagatara [Jakarta] potato. That is, in Holland what is known as an *aardappel*. It is baked and eaten. In the simplicity of its flavor it is like the *yamaimo*,[3] and in its sweetness, it is like the *satsumaimo*. Also, it has a delicious and nourishing stickiness and has no poison; so it can be used for daily meals. There are areas in Holland where the people live only on this. But it is not like the *satsumaimo*, which is sensitive to cold. Regardless of whether [it is planted in] a cold or a hot country, or whether in unfertile soil, one root will produce several clods.

I could not control my happiness at being given these two seeds. There could be nothing better in order to save the people from starvation and prevent them from becoming ill. I wanted to distribute [the seeds] in all directions; so I secretly consulted with my colleagues. They thought well of the idea and said, "Trying to save the people by erecting storehouses can help only one village or one commercial town. This is a fine and virtuous plan, which should reach the whole land for all time. We should not delay."

Accordingly, I had the things I had heard previously about cultivating and eating these crops written down and added to it selections from the explanations written in Dutch books to make a small pamphlet. I called it *Treatise on Two Things* and, together with the seeds, made it public.

---

2. *Apios fortunei*. A plant of the pulse family that grows in the mountainous areas of Japan.

3. *Dioscorea japonica*. A type of yam that is usually grated and used as a thickening agent.

Accordingly, incompetent man such as I am, bathing in the boundless good of the State, and enjoying my meals between bad years, I make this report for the unlikely event of an emergency, so that I may continue happily to avoid starvation.

> Written by Takano Yuzuru on the night of
> the Chrysanthemum Festival[4] at the
> Daikandō, Kaizaka, Kōjimachi, Edo

Thoughts About Two Things to Encourage Farming and Protect Against Poor Harvest

> By Zuikō[5] Takano Sensei
> Transcribed by Uchida (Kyō) Shikei[6]
> Edited by Fukuda (Sen) Sōtei and Yanagida (Shin) Teizō

Rapidly Maturing Buckwheat (Japanese names: hayasoba,[7] sandosoba,[8] Sōtei soba[9])

It is not clear where the first seeds of this buckwheat came from. In recent years, it has spread among the people and has been grown here and there. There is nothing in the stems and leaves to distinguish it from regular buckwheat, except that the grain is slightly bigger and it matures more quickly. For this reason, it ripens three times a year. Its Chinese name is not yet known. As a temporary name it is called *hayasoba* or *sandosoba.*

CULTIVATION. Like regular buckwheat, this buckwheat can be grown on infertile land. After waiting for the spring cold to subside and the land to thaw, at a time when there is no more frost to be seen, the soil should be plowed and the seeds sown in the same manner as regular buckwheat. The eighty-eighth day after the on-

---

4. Ninth of the ninth month.
5. Zuikō was one of Chōei's pen names.
6. Uchida Yatarō (1805–86). Uchida was one of Chōei's students of *rangaku.* See p. 38. Uchida also appends his own postscript to this work.
7. "Quick buckwheat."
8. "Three-times buckwheat."
9. Named after Fukuda Sōtei.

set of spring[10] is usually designated as the time for sowing, although in the eastern and northern provinces the spring cold is usually slower to ease and the frost more frequent; so it is better to plant the seeds a little later than this. Also, since buckwheat is very sensitive to cold, it can be killed by one overnight frost. Although this buckwheat can endure the cold a little more than other types, because it cannot survive the frost, it is important to observe the weather carefully when sowing the seeds. If the seedlings should be destroyed by frost, the soil should immediately be turned over, the seedlings buried in the earth to fertilize it, and new seeds planted. Usually the plants mature about 50 days after planting. (In cold areas, the time of maturation is a little later, but there is not a great difference). Thereupon, the crop should be harvested and used for seeds. The soil should be turned over again and seeds planted. These will again mature in about 50 days. However, this crop will be soft and difficult to use for seeds. Therefore, the first crop should be stored and used for seeds. After waiting for the next crop to mature, the soil should be turned over again and planted. Compared to the first two crops, it will be a little slower to mature, but nevertheless it will do so in no more than 60 days. In this way, generally within the space of a total of 150–60 days, three crops of buckwheat can be produced.

In our country, even in the lands to the north and east, there is nowhere that the ice does not thaw for five months of the year; so this buckwheat will always mature three times in the year. However, if the weather is unusual, and the spring cold is slow to finish and the autumn cold comes early, and one wants to be sure of it maturing three times, when the second round of seedlings are growing well, the space between the ridges should be lightly turned over and planted. When the time comes for harvesting, the third round of seedlings should be about two or three *sun*[11] tall and should be harvested early.

In this way, if the farmers grow this [buckwheat] and mix it with other things for their everyday meals, in one year they will have a surplus of two years' supply of grain, after two years they

---

10. A festival day.
11. One *sun* was 1.2 inches (3.03 cm).

will have four years' supply and after three years they will have six years' supply of grain. Is this not a large reserve for times when the harvest is poor? Similarly, if there is flooding in a particular year and the rice, wheat, and barley crops do not grow at all, and everywhere people are starving, there are at least one or two months in a year when the weather is normal. Therefore, even in times of terrible famine, this [buckwheat] can be grown and used as a food supply for the year. This is, after all, the reason why I think it is a great treasure for the whole land.

STORAGE. When the buckwheat is completely matured, it should be harvested and bleached in the sun to remove all moisture. Then it should be wrapped in a straw wrapper such as for rice or barley, or placed in a bucket and stored.

PREPARATION. The husk is removed in a hand mill and then the grain is steamed and eaten. Alternatively it is pounded to a fine flour and made into noodles or rice cakes. There are many other ways of eating buckwheat. It can also be made into *sake*. The method is described below.

BREWING OF *SAKE*. The Dutch use this grain to make beer. (This is the name of an alcoholic drink. It is slightly bitter). However, it is rarely made with this [grain] alone. Usually, another malt is added. To make it, grain from which the husk has been removed is taken and steamed. When it is cooked, it is put into a bowl and boiling water poured over. Barley malt and unrefined *sake* are added and stirred, after which it is covered tightly and placed in a warm place to ferment. When it bubbles and becomes alcoholic, the clear layer is poured off and used.

CHARACTER. Buckwheat has quite a lot of moisture compared to rice, barley, and wheat. For this reason, it is not a warming food by nature. Nevertheless, it is not lacking in nutrition, and in addition, it is easy to digest. Anyone can eat it and have no ill effects, but people who have a weak stomach should add to it something flavorsome and warming. Even so, if one has no other grain, it will do no harm to eat it on its own. In Friesland, one of the provinces of Holland, there is a place called Seehenouen[12] where it is very mountainous and the cold extremely severe. The mountain paths are very steep, and transportation is very inconvenient. The soil is sandy and stony, and nothing grows there except buckwheat, which the people use for food. This is proof [of the value of this grain].

VARIATIONS. The land to the north of Ezo[13] is generally called Siberia. This country is extremely cold; so there can be no question of [growing] rice. Even wheat and barley cannot mature there, and only buckwheat is grown. The stems and leaves are no different to the usual type, but the seed has jagged edges. It is said that the people there live entirely on this. This buckwheat must be able to withstand the frost. If [the grain] were imported to our country and grown here, it would mature four times a year. It is a great shame that we do not have the seeds. Nevertheless, it is not impossible to imagine[14] that the seeds could be growing of their own accord in the east and north of our country; so I include this as a guide for finding them.

OTHER. There is something similar to buckwheat, which is known in Holland as *suwarute uindo*.[15] Linnaeus (a great botanist of the West) calls it *Polygonum holees kaldachom*[16] in his book. It grows naturally by the roadsides and fences. Its stem is hard and can withstand the cold well. It is shaped like buckwheat and bears grain shaped like a prism, although quite small. It is probably similar to the wild buckwheat that grows here. The Dutch are also still unsure of its characteristics; so it is not yet used as a food. I would like to procure these seeds, as yet to no avail. If it has no poison and can be used like buckwheat, I think it would be of great bene-

---

12. Rendered from Chōei's *katakana*. I have been unable to confirm the place-name. See also the discussion on p. 124.

13. An old name for the northern island of Hokkaido.

14. Chōei has "it is impossible to imagine," but the words that follow do not allow this interpretation.

15. *Zwarte winde* (black bindweed).

16. *Polygonum foliis cordatis*.

fit to the country. I write this here and wait only for someone who knows to enlighten me.

Potato (*Japanese names:* jagataraimo,[17] kōshūimo,[18] chichibu-imo,[19] appura,[20] seidayuimo,[21] hasshōimo,[22] katsunenimo,[23] jumyōimo,[24] teizōimo;[25] *Dutch name:* aardappel)

The origin of this tuber is also unclear. It is said that it was imported to Kai and Shinano and grown from early times. When one considers that it is called *jagataraimo* or *appura* (which is a dialect of the hinterland and probably a corruption of *aardappel*), it would seem that it was brought by the Dutch. According to Dutch books, this potato grew originally in the West Indies, after which it was grown by the French and the English. After this it was introduced to the Dutch region. Also it is very common in America, where it seems the people who have emigrated there from Europe make this tuber the staple of their diet. That is, originally, this tuber came from the West Indies and America. It was grown for the first time in Holland about 1,600 years after the beginning of the era (this is about 200 years before the present year of 1836), and people still use it as their staple. Linnaeus (mentioned above) in his book writes about the three virtues of the potato. One, that it will flourish in areas with sandy and stony soil, where other grains will not grow. Two, it will not be damaged by strong winds, heavy rain, or long frosts. Third, it is easy to grow and does not require a lot of labor. Also, an inch of land will give the yield of a foot of land; so it is

---

17. Literally, "Jakarta tuber."
18. Kōshū is the old name for what is now Yamanashi prefecture.
19. Saitama prefecture.
20. A corruption of the Dutch.
21. Seidayu refers to Nakai Seidayu, *daikan* of Kai, who was active in promoting the cultivation of potatoes. See Murakami, "Kikin to daikan," p. 135.
22. Eight-*shō*-tuber. One *shō* was 1.92 quarts (1.8 liters). Eight was regarded as a lucky number.
23. Uncertain.
24. Literally, "lifespan" tuber.
25. Named after Yanagida Teizō.

also called a *hasshōimo*.[26] It certainly may be said to be a good crop for a bad year.

CULTIVATION. The potato should be sown around the eighty-eighth day after the beginning of spring. The earth should be plowed and the clods broken into little pieces. After that, two or three potatoes should be planted in one place and lightly covered with earth. The rest should also be planted in this way. The method is the same as for *satsumaimo*. Also, this potato is not particular about the type of soil in which it grows and will grow along the ridges of paddy fields, along the edge of roads, and in a mixture of sandy or stony soil; so it should be cultivated somewhere that it will not interfere with other crops. Also, it will endure the cold and can be grown in mountainous fields. Usually it will begin to sprout after about 30 days, after which it will grow a stem and tendrils. When the tendril is about two feet, leaving the end as is, the center part should be lightly covered with earth. From this place a new root and tendril will sprout. As the leaves and stems gradually increase in this way, one root will produce several clumps of potato. However, a new root will not produce as many clumps, and they will be small and watery. From the smaller root of the main root, several tens of clods will sprout, lined up like prayer beads. These will be fat and flavorsome and are considered the best. Also, these ones should be used as the seeds for the next year. In Holland, one root will yield 100 or 140–50 potatoes. However, in our country, the most one can get is usually from 40 to 70 potatoes. The leaves and stems gradually become taller and thicker, and the plant flowers in the autumn. After that, one waits until the plant dies off, and in cold areas the potatoes should be dug up and stored, while in warm areas the potatoes can be left in the ground and dug up when they are needed. In Holland, there are several methods for growing potatoes, of which two in particular are preferred. Therefore, I will summarize these below for reference.

The first method is in spring, to wait until the cold has completely gone and the ground has thawed, and then to plow the

---

26. See note 22.

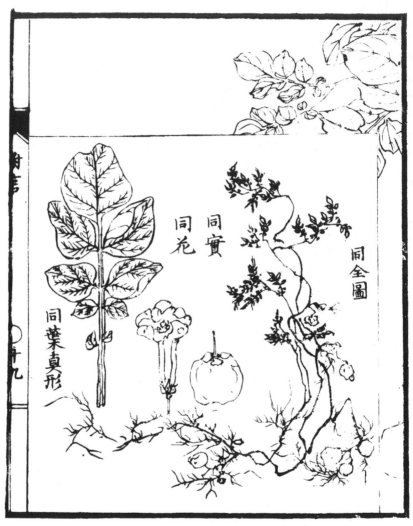

Fig. 1   Illustration of a potato, with insert, by Watanabe Kazan, from Takano
Chōei's *Kannō bikō nibutsukō*, 1836. Courtesy of Kyoto University Library.

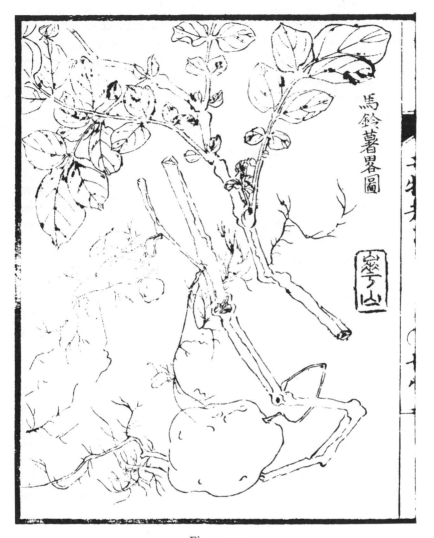

Fig. 1, cont.

earth, carefully breaking up the clumps and leveling the soil. Using a hoe, a ditch of about four *sun* in depth should be dug and the potatoes planted in groups of two or three, leaving a space of one *shaku*[27] between each group. However, big roots may be cut into two or three pieces. After that, the potatoes should be lightly covered with earth and smoothed over. Each row should be planted in this way. After they sprout leaves and stems, and flower in the autumn, the stems should be cut about four or five *sun* from the root, to prevent it from growing still more roots, and left to continue to grow. The stems should be used to feed horses and cattle, and after that, the roots dug up and stored.

The other method is to plant the potatoes as above, and when there are five or six sprouts coming out from each clump, after waiting for them to reach a length of about three *sun*, the sprouts should be lightly dug up by hand, and the thin root connecting it and the main root cut. In this way, each sprout should be taken, transferred to a new place and grown. After that, the main root should be taken out and turned over, and allowed to continue to grow. When the sprouts have once again grown to three *sun* in length, the new sprouts should be cut as in the beginning, and planted separately, leaving only one behind to be the main root. This method is extremely tedious, but if one wants several hundred potatoes from one root, then there is no better way than this. Otherwise, it does not differ from the above method. If one wishes to grow other kinds of vegetable or beans or barley at the same time, one should prepare the field in advance, leaving three *shaku* between each furrow, and plant the other crops in between. Fertilization should be done as for *satsumaimo*. It is also possible to fertilize at the time of planting. Also, it will do no harm if fertilizer is not used at all.

STORAGE. A hole two or three *shaku* deep should be dug in the earth, and the bottom laid with rice or barley straw, then the potatoes put in, and covered with another layer of straw and some earth, so as to prevent the cold from penetrating them. An opening should be made on one side and plugged with straw. When the po-

---

27. One *shaku* equals 0.994 foot (30.3 cm).

tatoes are required, they may be taken out through this opening. This is the method for storing them for the winter months in extremely cold climates. In warm areas, they may be kept in a corner of the garden or stable, and covered with a straw cover. If one wants to store them for several years, they should be peeled and sliced thinly, and left in the sun until completely dry, then wrapped in straw bags and stored.

PREPARATION. Fresh potatoes should be immediately boiled or steamed and used. If they are pungent, they should be soaked in lye until the acridity is removed. Dried potatoes should be soaked in warm water until soft and then boiled or steamed. The potatoes may be eaten alone, or mixed with rice, or made into hot soup, or used instead of green vegetables. There are a great many other ways of eating them according to one's taste. Also, there are methods of making the potatoes into flour or into an alcoholic spirit. The methods are as follows. (According to one account, the potato may also be used to make *konnyaku*.[28] The method is the same as for the *konnyaku* root.)

MAKING FLOUR. The method for making potato flour is the same as for making arrowroot or bracken-starch flour. The potatoes should be steeped in water for about twelve hours, taken out, and the skin removed. Then they should be steeped for another two to four hours and sliced thinly. The sliced potatoes are pounded in a mortar as if making rice cakes; then water is added to dilute it, before being filtered through a fine cloth. Put aside the milky water and pound the dregs in the mortar again, before adding water, stirring and filtering again, squeezing out the white liquid. The process should be repeated until the water is no longer cloudy. The liquid should be allowed to stand until the particles of potato settle on the bottom, then poured off. Water is again added, mixed, and allowed to stand, then tipped off. The process should be repeated until the liquid is colorless and tasteless. The liquid should be poured off, and [the remainder] allowed to dry in the

---

28. A kind of jelly made from the starch of the *konnyaku* (devil's tongue) plant.

sun or over a flame. This method is the same as for making arrow-root flour and bracken-starch flour, but the potato flour is said to be much better.

BREWING. Potatoes may also be made into *sake* in the same way as *satsumaimo*, but they cannot be made into unrefined *sake*. They should be distilled and made into hard liquor. Nevertheless, the character of this liquor is strong and aromatic, and it makes a fine spirit not unequal to millet brandy.[29] In Western books there are many ways to make this liquor. One method is to parboil the potatoes before taking them out and pounding them in a mortar until [the consistency of] a sticky rice cake. After that, they are diluted with boiling water until they look like a thin gruel. They are put in a bucket and left until the bubbling has stopped, the pure liquid has risen to the top and the dregs fallen to the bottom, before putting it in a distilling apparatus and making a distilled liquor. Another method is to peel the potatoes, and steam them until cooked. After that they are taken and pounded completely to a paste. Then the paste is diluted by pouring boiling water over, and millet or similar malt and unrefined *sake* are added and mixed well. While still warm, the mixture is placed in a bucket, tightly sealed, and left in a warm place to ferment. Every day, the lid is opened and the mixture is stirred once, before sealing it again. When it has developed a dry flavor, it is distilled and made into a hard liquor. Due to the pressures of work, I have not yet tested these methods carefully, and do not know which is the best. One day, after having tested it at home, I hope to expand on these details. The reason for my mentioning it in this book is merely to demonstrate that making distilled liquor from potatoes is another way to decrease the consumption of grains [for this purpose].

TYPES. There are three types of potato. One is white, one is red, and one is yellow. The red one grows big, but it is quite moist and the flavor is bland. The yellow one is a little acrid, so the white one is said to be better. In Holland, the white one in particular is grown and eaten. However, according to the nature of the soil, the

─────────

29. *Awamorishu*, 琉球酒.

red one might not grow big, and the white one might grow big instead, while the yellow one sometimes is not acrid; so it is difficult to say anything definite. After growing the potatoes in a particular soil, the nature of the soil should be clear; so one should at one's own discretion choose the type of potato most suitable.

NATURE. All three types [of potato] are nutritious and have no poison. Therefore, they should be used for daily meals. In addition, they will not become too sweet and acidify like *satsumaimo*. Because they have the advantage of greatly nourishing the stomach for a long time and allowing people to forget hunger, people in the West reserve their praise not for the *satsumaimo* but only for the potato. It is commonly said that because the potato is inimical to ink, those in the literary profession should not eat it, but this is wrong. A long time ago when pumpkins and *satsumaimo* were first grown, people thought that they were incompatible with fish or meat or that they would prevent people from writing with ink, and people everywhere were afraid and did not eat them very much. Now, people eat a great deal of them, even with fish and meat, and only then do they learn of the untruth of such sayings. Potatoes are another case of this. Previously, in the West, there was a time in Bolgonie [Boulogne] (a place in France), when it was said that potatoes caused scabies, and growing them was banned. However, since then people have eaten a great deal of them and there has been no record of any ill effects, which is proof of this. Ah, although all countries differ in their climate and customs, perhaps it is not only human sentiment that is the same!

The End

Postscript

A guest read this essay on potatoes and laughed, saying, "There was once an official who had a far-sighted plan. He knew the benefits of this tuber and decreed laws everywhere that it should be cultivated. But his plan was never carried out, and the seeds [that were to be planted] scarcely remain. Now, though one may tout the benefits [of potatoes] again as much as one likes, in the end, probably nothing will change."

I, Uchida Yatarō,[30] answered him, "Probably, since our country's soil is fertile and hundreds of grains flourish here, the people have enough to eat without growing other crops. In addition, in a usual year, if the people have a good crop, then they forget all about bad harvests and do not even store any of their good crops, let alone give any thought to other types. Although at the present time it is not clear why they do not plant these crops, perhaps this is where the reason lies. In addition, people do not know how to cook them, and there are various rumors about them being poisonous. Ah, what a shame it is! However, in recent years, we have suffered frequently from drought and flood, and now crop failure is severe. Among the people, there are many who are pale with hunger and have no time to give thought to the quality of their food. In addition, they regret the scarcity of their food stores. This autumn, it will be very easy for the people to adopt methods so that they might have a sufficient supply of food and to improve agriculture. This book explains in detail, from the way to cultivate and store [these foods] to their character and how to eat them. Also, it makes clear how to make flour and spirits and so on. Thus, even in an average year, people who grow these crops will reap many benefits. Even if one merely leaves them in infertile and abandoned soil, they will flourish of their own accord and may be harvested and eaten in a bad year. Indeed, there is no need for anyone in the country to starve to death. The nutritional advantages of these crops are incomparable to yams, flowering fern, and bracken. Once the people know of their benefits, surely they will rapidly turn to them like a rushing river."

The guest said only, "You should not worry about it so much," and left.

In the hours after that, I wrote this down as a postscript.

Uchida Yatarō
Scribe

---

30. See note 6.

Methods of Avoiding Epidemic Diseases

Preface

Famine and epidemic diseases are the most terrible of natural calamities, and they frequently occur at the same time. In this period of peace and prosperity, the administrators have a policy of charitable alms, and the people are thereby saved from starvation. Doctors have books about healing epidemic diseases; so the people need not die prematurely. Nevertheless, a method of avoiding these diseases has been previously unheard of. Before I got ill, I wrote a book called *Treatise on Contagious Diseases*, to which I attached an appendix on preventing epidemic diseases, but the editing was not yet finished. This winter, there had been signs of epidemic disease; so first of all I extracted the essential points [from the book] and had my student Takahashi Keisaku edit them, calling it *Methods of Avoiding Epidemic Diseases*. The reason I exclusively used the native script was so that people could easily be given a thorough understanding. Although this is too insignificant and trifling a composition to be given an audience, if people are thereby able to escape such suffering, surely this project may be of some benefit to society. A detailed account is contained in *Treatise on Contagious Diseases*; so people who wish to refer to this may do so.[1]

Written by Zuikō Takano Yuzuru Chōei, two days after the winter solstice, 1836, at Daikandō, Kaizaka, Kōjimachi, Edo

---

1. For further discussion of this document, see Chapter 4, pp. 124–32.

An Outline of Methods
of Avoiding Epidemic Diseases

At the times when epidemic fevers circulate, it is the same in both country and city; both noble and humble people are afraid of being infected and keep away from the sick, thinking that this is the way to avoid pestilence. This is not without reason, but essentially at times when epidemic fevers are rampant, they occur because there is a different kind of bad air in the land; so sometimes even if one is not infected immediately as a result of visiting someone sick, one can unintentionally be exposed to this atmosphere and spontaneously develop the disease. Most important, therefore, is that people should take care of their health in order not to catch the disease.

There are very many methods of preventative medicine: using an emetic medicine, or using a medicine to tone the stomach, bleeding, or using a purgative medicine. All of these are effective. However, using a purgative to clean the bowels and remove stagnation is the best method of avoiding an epidemic disease. For this medicine, take two *monme*[2] of Chinese rhubarb,[3] one *monme* of *haōen*[4] (explained below), and one *monme* of white soap (explained below). First, make a powder from the rhubarb and *haōen*, mix in the soap, and use starch to make into balls. Five *fun*[5] in weight should be used in one day, to effect about two bowel movements per day. The preparation should be used for three or four days in a row. If, for example, in rural areas these medicines cannot be purchased, then out of necessity, two *monme* of rhubarb and one *monme* of saltpeter should be made into a powder and mixed with starch to

---

2. A *monme* was equivalent to 0.1325 ounce (3.75 grams).

3. *Rheum officinale*. Used as a general eliminant and tonic for the digestive system; recommended for women's diseases and fevers. See Smith, *Chinese Materia Medica*, p. 375.

4. This term could not be translated. Literally, the characters 覇王塩 mean "hegemon salt." Judging from the procedure Chōei describes, it was probably some kind of inert ash. He may well have discovered it simply in the process of his own experimentation. In any case, the soap and Chinese rhubarb with which he mixed it for this purgative medicine were sufficiently potent for a powerful purge (Nathan Sivin, personal communication, May 2000).

5. One tenth of a *monme*, i.e., 0.01325 ounce (0.375 grams).

form balls of medicine. It can also be used in a powdered form. Alternatively, *sankōgan*[6] or *kyūkōsan*[7] may be used. Depending on the constitution of the patient, use five or six *fun*.

By using this method, as long as there are no other unhealthy conditions, in most cases, one will not succumb to an epidemic fever. Even if one does happen to be infected, the symptoms will be slight, and the disease will not lead to death. The likely reason for the prevalence of epidemic fevers after a famine is that the poor quality of food causes dirt to stagnate in the belly and the stomach to weaken; so what begins as a slight cold may finally develop into an epidemic disease. There is a very reasonable explanation for this, which I treat in detail in my book *Treatise on Contagious Diseases*, but since this is not something that the average person needs to know, I will omit this. In any case, one should make the cleaning of the digestive system one's first priority. For all that, having too many bowel movements is also damaging to the stomach and intestines; so after having purged the bowels one or two times in the month, one should take two or three doses of the following infusion to tone the digestive organs. To make it, take two large scoops of giant hyssop,[8] a small scoop each of rose banksia and longan,[9] and a large scoop of Chinese peony,[10] steep them in water and use.

Also, because epidemic diseases occur in places where the atmosphere is gloomy, one should take care to keep the inside of

---

6. A mixture of skullcap (*Scutellaria macrantha*), Chinese rhubarb (*Rheum officinale*), and goldthread (*Coptis teeta*) mixed with honey; used as a tonic. See Smith, *Chinese Materia Medica*, p. 330.

7. Probably a mixture of powdered *Conioselinum univittatum* and Chinese rhubarb.

8. *Lophanthus rugosis*. The branches and leaves are used in medicine. It is said to relieve flatulence and aid digestion; used in the treatment of cholera, as a mouthwash, and for morning sickness. See Smith, *Chinese Materia Medica*, p. 247.

9. *Nephelium longana*. A plant related to the lichee. The fruits are supposed to increase the mental faculties and act upon the spleen. They are also used as a worm treatment and as an antidote to poison. The seeds are used for excessive perspiration. See Smith, *Chinese Materia Medica*, p. 282.

10. *Paeonia albiflora*. It is used widely in Chinese medicine as a general tonic. It is said to relieve pain and flatulence and work as a diuretic; works on the spleen, stomach, and intestines, and helps with hemorrhage; also recommended for diseases of pregnancy. See Smith, *Chinese Materia Medica*, p. 300.

one's house clean and free of dust. The reason why there are many epidemic fevers in rural areas is because the front of the courtyard and so on is not cleaned properly and the inside of the rooms is gloomy; so even if there is no poisonous fever there in the first place, it spontaneously develops. Even in Edo, it is due to the presence of a gloomy atmosphere that there are always epidemic fevers in places such as the servants' quarters, *osukuigoya*,[11] or in prison, even at times when there are no such diseases in general circulation. Also in places like large trading houses, where several people eat and sleep lined up like fish scales in a narrow space, or in backstreet houses with only one entrance, there is a great deal of epidemic fever, whereas in spacious residences there is little epidemic fever. This depends on whether or not there is a gloomy atmosphere. Therefore, one should take special care to have a window in bedrooms and in living rooms in order to create good ventilation. According to the customs of our country, not only with regard to epidemic fevers, but also in general, when we have a feverish illness we use heavy bedclothes and shut the windows tight, or we place a screen around in order to keep out any draft. However, to think it is good to do nothing but sweat is a terrible mistake. This can turn a slight illness into a serious one. Please understand this point well, and be sure to provide good ventilation so as to remove stale dirty air and bring in fresh clean air from outside.

A good method of changing the air is: in winter, close the windows and doors of the patient's bedroom, and place a large brazier in which a fire has been lit [inside the room] to make it warm. Then the doors and windows should suddenly be opened, and in so doing the stale air will go outside, and the fresh air from outside will come in, allowing an exchange of old for new. After that, the brazier should be removed, and the door closed. Usually for a feverish illness, this procedure should be carried out three or four times a day. In the summer time, it is not necessary to use a fire. One should make sure that a little breeze is able to enter the room, and that it is slightly cool. In addition, it is not advisable for many people to crowd into the room to care for the patient, as it causes the atmo-

---

11. *Osukuigoya* were relief stations set up by authorities during times of famine or disaster. They provided food and medicines for the needy.

sphere to become bad. Unnecessary people should not be allowed to enter the room. However, if for some unavoidable reason, there are many people in the room, one should carry out the above method several times to change the air. Even so, it is not advisable for the room to be so drafty as to make the patient feel cold. One should use one's discretion and keep the temperature comfortable.

It goes without saying that epidemic fever may infect the caregiver and even sometimes spread to the surrounding area. Thus it has been a custom since old times in our country for a caregiver to put camphor, musk, or something with an aromatic, sharp smell in the nose and to burn aloes or *okera*[12] in the next room. Near the patient, *okera*, dried orange peel, and juniper tree are burned as a matter of course; even things like dried cuttlefish are used in order to avoid the poisonous air. It seems to me that these are not good methods. They have no benefit and do a great deal of damage; so they should not be employed. There are several good methods of using inhalations to avoid disease. One method is to moisten the end of a straw broom with vinegar and sweep it about, sprinkling the walls and doors. In an earthen bowl place some Borneo camphor vinegar (described below) and heat it over a low heat, filling the room with the steam. One should sniff it every now and then. Another method is to place a pot over the hearth and fill it with ashes and sand, then take a clay jar and bury it half way in the sand mixture. Fill the jar with sea salt. When the ashes, sand, and salt are warm, pour sulfuric acid (explained below) over the salt, causing smoke to arise and fill the room. Usually, for a room the size of 40 *tatami* mats, 78 *monme* of sea salt and 65 *monme* of sulfuric acid are sufficient. Please adjust the amounts in this proportion according to the size of the room. Although both methods are good for controlling the epidemic poison and preventing infection, there are some who dislike the vinegary atmosphere or some who hate the camphorous air, making it difficult to use these methods. Some people choke or start coughing as soon as they are exposed to the smoke and damage their lungs; so although this may be carried out

---

12. *Atractylis ovata.* A plant that grows in dry, mountainous areas, the young shoots may be eaten as a food, and the dried stems are used as a tonic for the stomach and bladder. It is said to have the power to drive away evil spirits.

in places such as a bedroom where someone has died from epidemic fever or in an empty room where no one has lived for a long time, it cannot be used in rooms and bedrooms where people are. For these reasons, the following method is best. Take some fine sand and place it in an earthen pot over the hearth, until the moisture is removed. Then take a small pottery *sake* cup, and bury it halfway in the sand. Fill it with about four *monme* of powdered saltpeter and warm it a little. Close the windows and doors; take about four *monme* of sulfuric acid and pour it over the saltpeter. Stir it frequently with glass tongs (do not use metal tongs) and allow the smoke to rise. This vapor has a remarkable ability to control epidemic poison and does not harm the breathing. It also has the advantage of cooling fever; so everywhere one thinks poisonous air might be stagnating, this bowl should be placed, and the mixture vaporized. In a bad case of epidemic fever, one should use this method to vaporize the bedroom two or three times a day. If in the countryside, due to the shortage of materials, one is unable to carry out this procedure, one should, if necessary, burn a touch of saltpeter over a fire or burn sparklers and fill the room with the smoke.

Information for Caregivers or Those Visiting People with Epidemic Fevers

One, saliva has a propensity to be easily contaminated with poison; so when near the patient, one should be careful not to swallow it, but to spit it out. Two, one should not care for the patient when very hungry, but after one has eaten. In cases where it cannot be helped, then one should at least drink a little *sake*. Three, one should apply Borneo camphor vinegar to the inside of the nose. Orpiment[13] should not be used. Four, if the patient is sweating profusely and the room smells sweaty, the door should be opened and a fresh breeze allowed in. Five, the patient's clothes should sometimes be changed, washed, and clean ones put on. The bedclothes should also be shaken out and the room cleaned several times a day. Six, be careful to avoid extreme temperatures in the patient's room. Seven, do not allow a lot of people into the room,

---

13. A mineral form of arsenic trisulfide.

especially if the room is small. Eight, caregivers and visitors should take a bath or wash every day, and change into clean clothes. Utensils used by the patient should be carefully rinsed. For making medicinal tea, a pottery bowl is preferable. Nine, epidemic fevers are frightening, but one should not be too frightened. Excessive fear can make one more susceptible to the disease or make it worse once infected. Ten, do not sleep in the same bed as the patient.

If these ten rules are followed and the medicines and methods explained above are used, then in many cases infection will not occur. Therefore, do not be afraid to care for or visit those you love. In country areas, there are times when even family and close friends stop visiting those with epidemic diseases, and they simply sit back and watch the patient die. This is a sad thing, and the reason why it happens is because people do not know how to prevent the disease.

What to Do After People Have Recovered from Epidemic Diseases or After They Have Died

When a patient dies from an epidemic fever, the body should quickly be prepared and buried. However, people who die from epidemic fever sometimes come back to life when they are exposed to the vapors of the earth; so be well aware of this and continue to watch out even after burial. The chopsticks and clothes used by the sick person should be washed without delay to remove the poison, and the clothes should be worn after permeating with incense. After recovery or death, the patient's room should be well cleaned. During the day, the windows and doors should be opened to change the air. A vase may be filled with water and flowers and placed in a sunny position in the room to fill the air with their fresh atmosphere. Alternatively, the smoke arising from a mixture of sea salt and sulfuric acid, as described above, may be used.

A Good Method of Protecting Against Epidemic Diseases and Stopping Their Spread

In a certain faraway country, at a time when epidemic disease was rampant, not only kings and noblemen as a matter of course but wealthy farmers, merchants, and other powerful persons too supplied the funds to build a new hospital. Whenever someone came down with an epidemic fever, they were quickly transferred there, a doctor was called, and nursing staff supplied to care for the patient; so that the disease was stopped from spreading to others. Probably, it is due to the isolation of smallpox victims that there are some places in our country where there is now no smallpox. This method is extremely important for preventing epidemic disease. Epidemic fevers are far more damaging to people than famine. The healing of epidemic fevers with medicine is only secondary. What I hope to do is to treat the cause, and this is, in short, the reason why I am writing of this method of avoiding epidemics.

How to Make Haōen

Take equal quantities of sulfur and saltpeter, and pound them to a powder, mixing well. Light a flame in a pottery bowl and add the powder little by little with a spoon. After doing so, and after the flame has extinguished, take the burnt remains and put them in an earthen bowl, add water, and gently simmer. When the dregs have all dissolved into the water and a skin has formed on the surface, remove from the heat and strain through a fine cloth. Leave to cool. Take the salt that hardens and congeals on the bottom of the dish and around the edges, and use. This is *haōen*.[14]

About Soap

Soap is called *shabon* in Japanese. There are three types: two types of white soap and one amber-colored product. One type of white soap comes from Holland, and the other comes from China. The latter is inferior and cannot be used for internal medicine. The former one, from Holland, is said to be white in color and square in shape. It should be used internally. If this is not available, then the amber-colored soap should be used. This, too, comes from Holland. It is also made in Japan, although the quality is inferior. It may be used to remove dirt but cannot be used internally.[15]

---

14. See note 4.
15. Soap was used internally as a purgative.

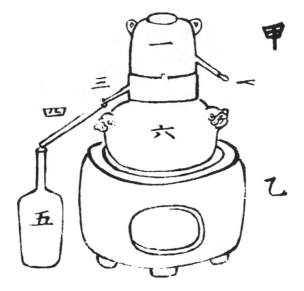

Fig. 2 Illustration of a still, from Takano Chōei's *Hieki yōhō*,
1836. Courtesy of Kyoto University Library.

How to Make Refined Borneo Camphor Vinegar

Take two gō[16] of strong vinegar and four *monme* of Borneo camphor. First, pound the Borneo camphor into a fine powder. Gradually add the vinegar and mix well. Next, put it into a distiller as pictured below, and treat as if making a hard spirit. Catch the distilled liquid in a glass bottle. Usually about five *shaku*[17] will be collected. When the flavor becomes weak, take the bottle away and plug it with beeswax or a seal made from hardened hair oil so that its potency cannot escape, and store.

Explanation of the Diagram

甲 is a picture of the whole still (see Fig. 2). It is best to use one from pottery. 乙 is the bath. The coals should be as soft as possible. 一 is where one puts the water, and when it is hot, the plug, 二

16. A gō equals 0.384 pint (0.18 liters).
17. One *shaku* is one-tenth of a gō, i.e., 0.384 pint (0.018 liters).

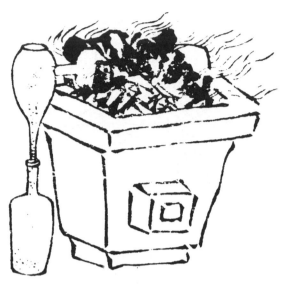

Fig. 3 Illustration of a still, from Takano Chōei's *Hieki yōhō*,
1836. Courtesy of Kyoto University Library.

should be removed and the water let out. Replace the plug and fill
with cold water. This process should be repeated several times. 二
is the place where the water is drained away. Be sure to plug it. 三
is where the droplets of distilled liquid emerge. 四 is a bamboo
pipe. 五 is a glass bottle. 六 is the base of the distiller and is where
the Borneo camphor should be placed.

How to Make Sulfuric Acid

Take a heat-resistant bottle (a rustic *sake* bottle is good), paint it
with plaster and allow to dry (see Fig. 3). Make some ferrous sul-
fate into a rough powder, and roast it to remove the moisture. Fill
the bottle to about seven parts with this. Place the mouth of the
bottle inside the side of another small *sake* bottle into which a hole
has been made. Paint the join with plaster. Place the bottle at a
slight angle as in the picture, over a small portable clay stove, pile
up the coals all over it, and cook over a strong heat. Drops of liquid will come out of the mouth of the small bottle. At first they
will be pale in color and have no taste. They should be thrown
away as they come out. Usually, after about two hours, the matter

that comes out will be like smoke. People will cough when they are exposed to it, and it is acidic and sour in taste. At this point, a Dutch glass bottle should be placed over the mouth of the small bottle (Japanese bottles are difficult to use), and the join painted with plaster, so that the gas cannot escape and falls in drops into the bottle. Coals should be added throughout so that the fire does not lose its intensity. If the large bottle should break and smoke should escape, it should be mended with plaster. Usually on a spring day, it should be baked from morning until evening. When no more smoke comes out of the mouth of the bottle, remove the glass bottle and seal with beeswax or a plug made from hair oil to ensure that its potency will not escape, and store. This method is extremely abbreviated. Please see the book called *Nibutsukō*[18] for a detailed explanation.

Appendix

Using the above methods, many people are able to avoid epidemic fevers. However, due to their constitutions, some people are unable to escape them, and in remote rural areas, where there is a shortage of doctors, they knowingly neglect their treatment. In some cases, what begins as a minor case, which would have been easily curable, becomes worse and difficult to heal. For this reason, I will now outline below a method of treatment that even a lay person is able to use, so that from the beginning, the illness may be treated quickly and without error. If I were to make a comparison, in order to remove grasses and trees, one must pull them out before the roots grow deep and the branches and leaves flourish. In the same way, illness should be treated before it gathers in strength. However, it is difficult for a lay person to know whether or not the disease is an epidemic fever. Thus, if there is epidemic fever in the vicinity, and the patient complains of heavy limbs, headache, feels a terrible chill, and breaks out in a sweat, then it should be thought of as an epidemic fever and the following medicine administered promptly.

---

18. The text has *Nabutsukō*. I have taken this title to be *Nibutsukō*, Chōei's pamphlet on famine relief. The extant version of this pamphlet, however, does not contain a detailed explanation of distillation.

An Outline for Treating the Epidemic Fevers That Occur After Famine

Epidemic fevers differ slightly according to the year and the season in which they occur. In addition, even though exposed to the same poison, people's symptoms will vary according to their constitutions. Therefore, it is difficult to prescribe a definite treatment. However, many of the epidemic diseases that are prevalent after famine have their origin in impurities in the stomach and intestine and have similar symptoms; so here I will outline their treatment.

First of all, before the patient has lost too much strength, the impurities should be removed from the stomach. An emetic is good for this. Among emetic medicines, ipecacuanha (from Holland) is especially good. The dosage for an adult is about three *fun* and three *rin*[19] at a time. Also for ipecacuanha wine (the same as above), from two to four *rin* may be used. Gourd stems cause severe dizziness and should not be used. In general, after the patient takes the emetic and becomes nauseous, three or four glasses of lukewarm salty water should be given to induce vomiting. Patients who have fur on the tongue should use an emetic as quickly as possible. If this medicine is hard to obtain, then the patient should drink several glasses of lukewarm salty water and put the end of a chicken wing in the throat to cause vomiting. After vomiting, the purgative medicine mentioned above should be used and the bowels emptied two or three times. After that, dissolve one *fun* of saffron in warm water and drink all at once. Usually if the impurities are removed from the stomach and intestines in this way, a mild case will be cured by this alone, and even in severe cases there will be few that end in death.

However, if the symptoms are not relieved, fill a tub or large bucket with water that is hotter than usual, add one *gō* of powdered mustard and stir well. The patient should wear thick clothes, and, rolling up his trousers, place both legs in this hot water, bathing half the body up to below the groin. The water should be hotter than usual, and the bath should be finished after about thirty minutes

---

19. One tenth of a *fun*.

when there is sweat over the entire body. Wipe the legs, put the patient to bed, and cover with thick bedclothes. Use ten *monme* of elderflowers[20] in three *gō* of water, boil it down to one *gō* and use this all at once to induce sweat. Do not use a medicine made with *katsura*[21] bark to induce sweating. Usually, this method should be used twice a day. If the patient is very thirsty, squeeze a bitter orange or a lemon, add sugar, and mix with hot water. This may be given several times a day. If the patient does not sweat, take about five *monme* each of honey and rice vinegar, mix together and decoct. Stir occasionally, and stop when it has boiled down to about six or seven *monme*. This should be given two or three times a day. This medicine is also excellent for coughing and laryngitis.

For severe headache, place about five or six leeches on the temple to suck the blood. Alternatively, scarify the area with a needle and draw blood by cupping. If this does not alleviate the pain, add some vinegar to warm water, then add three *monme* of saltpeter. Soak a hand towel in the bath, wring, and place it on the temples and forehead to warm the head with the steam. Or, take three *rin* of camphor and five *bu* of saltpeter and make into a fine powder. Add wheat flour to make a starchy ball. This [medicine] may be used twice. If the patient cannot sweat, dissolve three *fun* of powdered borax in four *monme* of strong vinegar, and administer all at once. In most cases, the patient will sweat. If the patient does not begin to sweat after one administration, it may be given two or three times.

For insomnia, dissolve one *fun* of saffron in warm water and give the liquid a little at a time. Also, epidemic fevers that are caused by impurities in the stomach and intestines weaken the stomach itself; so after using emetic and purgative medicines, continue to give the following infusion once a day. Take two large scoops of giant hyssop, a small scoop of rose banksia, a small scoop of gentian,[22] and a large scoop of barley. Mix together and infuse briefly in water.

---

20. *Sambucus racemosa*. This emetic must be used carefully. The juice is used for broken bones, sprains, colds, and tooth decay. The bark is used for dropsy, fevers, and a delayed afterbirth. The leaves are used for ague. See Smith, *Chinese Materia Medica*, p. 393.

21. *Cercidiphyllum japonicum*.

22. Refers to several species of *gentiana*. It was prescribed for fevers, rheumatism, noxious odors, abnormal discharges, and feebleness in general; used locally

Pains in the stomach and nausea in many cases come from intestinal worms. If these symptoms are present, take two large scoops of Corsican weed,[23] a medium scoop of Chinese rhubarb, a small scoop of anise,[24] and a large scoop of barley. Mix together, boil in water, and administer. If the chest is constricted and painful, take seven *monme* of hollyhock roots,[25] five *monme* of winter chrysanthemum,[26] six *monme* of elderflowers, put in a large bag and place in seven *gō* of water. Boil it down to five *gō*, then add five *shaku* of vinegar. Close tightly, and use it to warm the chest and stomach with the steam.

If care is taken from the beginning to treat illness promptly using the above methods, most cases will be cured. However, these are the simplest methods of treating the diseases that are prevalent after eating a poor diet in famine years and are only medicines that can be used by lay persons without harm. They will not cure all epidemic diseases. Nevertheless, these methods, if used in the early stages of any epidemic fever, have a helpful effect; so whatever the disease, do not be afraid to use them promptly. It should be possible to cure slight cases immediately and completely. It is not my urgent business now to write about the treatment for other epidemic fevers, and it is not possible to write in detail in this small book, so I will omit this here and leave it for another book. Please do not condemn me, dear readers, for the deficiencies.

Edited by pupil Takahashi Keisaku, of Jōmō

----

for skin diseases and ulcers; recommended as a treatment for worms, nocturnal sweating, eye diseases, and blood in the urine. See Smith, *Chinese Materia Medica*, pp. 186–87.

23. *Diginea simplex*. A kind of seaweed.

24. *Pimpinella anisum*. A warming medicine, prescribed for flatulence. See Smith, *Chinese Materia Medica*, p. 331.

25. *Althea rosea*. According to Smith, the parts of the plant used are the shoots, which are used for their regulative and stomachic properties and in fevers, labor, and dysentery, and the rootstock and seeds, which are used as a diuretic and applied to ulcers. See Smith, *Chinese Materia Medica*, p. 33.

26. *Chrysanthemum indicum*. Commonly used in the treatment of blood circulation, colds, headaches, inflamed eyes, and for general vitality. See Smith, *Chinese Materia Medica*, p. 107.

Each time there is a great disaster, it is followed by epidemic disease. In the spring following the disaster of Tenmei 6 [1786], it is said that ten times more people died from epidemic disease than of starvation. This year, the famine has been much the same as it was in Tenmei 6, and epidemic diseases have been increasing steadily. Takano-ō[27] laments this and has written this little book in which he gives details of how to avoid and heal these diseases. Epidemics circulate and are avoided and, if unavoidable, are healed. In the midst of disaster, the book has a wide-ranging power to relieve suffering, like a boat to rely on when the bridge is broken. On the joyful occasion of its printing, five days after the winter solstice of 1836, Hagura[28] wrote [the following postscript].

Uchida Kyō, scribe[29]

In this year of 1836, there has been a bad harvest, and in every province, there is famine. Once a wise person said that perhaps it is in the nature of things that diseases follow immediately after a famine. For this reason, Takano-ō humbly wrote *Treatise on Two Things for the Relief of Famine*, and *Treatise on Contagious Diseases*, which are urgently needed and erudite books. When saving lives is urgent, one does not wait from morning until the evening; so he wrote about the methods of avoiding epidemic diseases as the first step in this process. It is indeed praiseworthy to hope to save the common people from sinking into early death. With sighs of admiration, I write this brief afterword.

Read three days after the beginning of the second severest cold, 1836, by a student of medicine.[30]

The End

---

27. A term of respect.

28. This Hagura was probably the Confucian scholar and educator Hagura Geki (1790–1862). He is believed to have associated with Watanabe Kazan and was employed for a time as the Bakufu intendant of government territory in Kōzuke, among other provinces. See Satō, *Yōgakushi kenkyū josetsu*, p. 197.

29. See p. 38.

30. Around January 8 of the following year, by the Western calendar.

Books by Takano Zuikō Sensei[31]

Fundamentals of Medicine, vol. 1 (five books, special edition)

Fundamentals of Medicine, vol. 2 (seven books, soon to be published)

Zuikō's Hackneyed Work (ten books, soon to be published)

A Brief History of Holland (seven volumes, soon to be published)

Western Magazine (fifteen books, soon to be published)

A Compilation of Strange Utensils (ten volumes, soon to be published)

Treatise on Contagious Diseases, including Methods of Avoiding Epidemic Diseases (two books, special edition)

Treatise on Two Things (one volume, carving completed)[32]

The Steward, Daikandō[33]
Izumiya Kichibei Bookstore,
opposite Shiba Shinmei, Edo

---

31. This appears to be an advertisement for the Izumiya Kichibei bookstore, which was located, as indicated, opposite the Shiba Shinmei Shrine. The bookstore was a member of the *minami* group of booksellers, which consisted of Edo-rather than Kyoto-based businesses. The store may be found on a register of this group from 1809. See Konta, *Edo no hon'yasan*, p. 89.

32. With the exception of the second volume of *Fundamentals of Medicine*, all the works labeled as forthcoming do not appear to have been completed, a sad indication of the way in which Chōei's career was cut off in its prime by his untimely imprisonment.

33. Daikandō was the name of Chōei's school.

Reference Matter

Works Cited

Abiko, Bonnie. "Watanabe Kazan: The Man and His Times." PhD diss., Princeton University, 1982.

Agricultural Bureau, Department of Agriculture and Commerce. *Outlines of Agriculture*. Tokyo: 1910.

Amano Hiroshi. *Kusuri bunka ōrai*. Tokyo: Seiabō, 1992.

Amino Yoshihiko. *Zoku Nihon no rekishi o yominaosu*. Tokyo: Chikuma shobō, 1996.

Aoki Toshiyuki. "Itō Chūtai hisshya 'Takano shi sōbyōron.'" In *Jitsugakushi kenkyū*, ed. Jitsugakushiryō kenkyūkai, pp. 253–68. Kyoto: Shibunkaku, 1993.

———. "Sōmō no rangaku." In *Bunka no taishūka*. Nihon no kinsei 14, ed. Takeuchi Makoto, pp. 219–68. Tokyo: Chūō kōronsha, 1993.

———. *Zaison rangaku no kenkyū*. Kyoto: Shibunkaku, 1998.

Arakawa Hidetoshi. *Saigai no rekishi*. Tokyo: Nihon rekishi shinsho, 1967.

Ariyoshi, Sawako. *The Doctor's Wife*. Translated by Wakako Hironaka and Ann Siller Kostant. Tokyo: Kodansha International, 1978.

Bailey, L. H. *The Standard Cyclopedia of Horticulture*. 3 vols. New York: Macmillan, 1930.

Bartholomew, James. *The Formation of Science in Japan*. New Haven: Yale University Press, 1989.

Beasley, W. G. *Great Britain and the Opening of Japan, 1834–1858*. London: Luzac, 1951.

Benedict, Carol. *Bubonic Plague in Nineteenth-Century China*. Stanford: Stanford University Press, 1996.

Beukers, Harm [Harmen]. "The Fight Against Smallpox in Japan: The Value of Western Medicine Proved." In *Red-Hair Medicine: Dutch-Japanese Medical Relations*, ed. Harm Beukers, A. M. Luyendijk-Elshout, M. E. van Opstall, and F. Vos, pp. 59–77. Amsterdam: Rodopi, 1991.

———. *The Mission of Hippocrates in Japan*. Amsterdam: Four Centuries of Netherlands-Japan Relations, 1998.

Bourke, Austin. *"The Visitation of God"? The Potato and the Great Irish Famine*. Dublin: Lilliput Press, 1993.

Bowers, John. *Western Medical Pioneers in Feudal Japan*. Baltimore: Johns Hopkins Press, 1970.

———. *When the Twain Meet*. Baltimore: Johns Hopkins University Press, 1980.

Casal, U. A. "Acupuncture, Cautery and Massage in Japan." *Folklore Studies* 21 (1962): 221–35.

Chaiklin, Martha. *Cultural Commerce and Dutch Commercial Culture*. Leiden: Research School CNWS, Leiden University, 2003.

Cuncliffe, Barry. *The City of Bath*. Gloucester, Eng.: Allan Sutton, 1986.

Davey, Basiro; Tim Halliday; and Mark Hirst, eds. *Human Biology and Health: An Evolutionary Approach*. 3rd ed. Buckingham, Eng.: Open University Press, 2001.

de Bary, Wm. Theodore. "Introduction." In *Principle and Practicality*, ed. Wm. Theodore de Bary and Irene Bloom, pp. 1–36. New York: Columbia University Press, 1979.

De Candolle, Alphonse. *Origin of Cultivated Plants*. 2nd ed. New York: Hafner Publishing, 1959.

Digby, Anne. *Making a Medical Living : Doctors and Patients in the English Market for Medicine, 1720–1911*. Cambridge, Eng.: Cambridge University Press, 1994.

Dobson, Mary. *Contours of Death and Disease in Early Modern England*. Cambridge, Eng.: Cambridge University Press, 1997.

Fujikawa Yū. *Isha no fūzoku, meishin*. Fujikawa Yū chosaku shū, vol. 3, Kyoto: Shibunkaku, 1975.

———. *Nihon igakushi kōyō*. Tokyo: Heibonsha, 1974.

Fukui Hidetoshi, Miyasaka Masahide, and Tokunaga Hiroshi. *Siebold's Japan*. Nagasaki: Siebold Memorial Museum, 2001.

Gluck, Carol. "The Invention of Edo." In *Mirror of Modernity: Invented Traditions of Modern Japan*, ed. Stephen Vlastos, pp. 262–84. Berkeley: University of California Press, 1998.

Goodman, Grant. *Japan: The Dutch Experience*. London: Athlone Press, 1986.

Greene, David C. "Life of Takano Nagahide." *Transactions of the Asiatic Society of Japan* 41 (1913): 390–492.

Grilli, Peter, and Dana Levy. *Pleasures of the Japanese Bath*. New York: Weatherhill, 1992.

Grist, Norman, et al. *Diseases of Infection: An Illustrated Textbook*. Oxford: Oxford University Press, 1987.

Gunma ken shi hensan iinkai, ed. *Gunma ken shi*. Tsūshihen 6. Maebashi: Gunma ken, 1992.

Hamlin, Christopher. "Predisposing Causes and Public Health in Early Nineteenth-Century Medical Thought." *Social History of Medicine* 5, no. 1 (1992): 43–70.

Haneveld, G.T. "The Introduction of Acupuncture into Western Medicine: The Influence of Japanese and Dutch Physicians." In *Red-Hair Medicine: Dutch-Japanese Medical Relations*, ed. Harm Beukers, A. M. Luyendijk-Elshout, M. E. van Opstall, and F. Vos, 51–58. Amsterdam: Rodopi, 1991.

Hanley, Susan. *Everyday Things in Premodern Japan*. Berkeley: University of California Press, 1997.

———. "Tokugawa Society: Material Culture, Standard of Living, and Life-Styles." In *The Cambridge History of Japan*, vol. 4, *Early Modern Japan*, ed. J. W. Hall, pp. 660–705. Cambridge, Eng.: Cambridge University Press, 1991.

Hanley, Susan, and Kozo Yamamura. *Economic and Demographic Change in Preindustrial Japan, 1600–1868*. Princeton: Princeton University Press, 1977.

Harootunian, H. D. "Late Tokugawa Culture and Thought." In *The Cambridge History of Japan*, vol. 5, *The Nineteenth Century*, ed. Marius Jansen, pp. 168–258. Cambridge, Eng.: Cambridge University Press, 1989.

Hattori Toshirō. *Edo jidai igakushi no kenkyū*. Tokyo: Yoshikawa kōbunkan, 1978.

Heibonsha, ed. *Nihonshi daijiten*. 7 vols. Tokyo: Heibonsha, 1992–94.

Hirata Atsutane. "Kodō Taii." In *Hirata Atsutane*. Nihon no meicho, vol. 24, ed. Sagara Tōru, pp. 83–155. Tokyo: Chūō kōronsha, 1972.

Howell, David. "Social Disorder and Moral Reform in Late Tokugawa Japan." Paper presented at the Japanese Studies Association of Australia Biennial Conference, Central Queensland University, Rockhampton, 1999.

Hyams, Edward. *Plants in the Service of Man*. London: J. M. Dent and Sons, 1971.

Inkster, Ian. "Marginal Men: Aspects of the Social Role of the Medical Community in Sheffield, 1790–1850." In *Health Care and Popular Medicine in Nineteenth Century England*, ed. John Woodward and David Richards, pp. 128–63. London: Croom Helm, 1977.

Jannetta, Ann Bowman. *Epidemics and Mortality in Early Modern Japan*. Princeton: Princeton University Press, 1987.

———. "Famine Mortality in Nineteenth-Century Japan: The Evidence from a Temple Death Register." *Population Studies* 46 (1992): 427–43.

———. "The Introduction of Jennerian Vaccination in Nineteenth-Century Japan." *Japan Foundation Newsletter* 23, no. 2 (1995): 6–9.

Jansen, Marius. "Japan in the Early Nineteenth Century." In *The Cambridge History of Japan*, vol. 5, *The Nineteenth Century*, ed. Marius Jansen, pp. 50–115. Cambridge, Eng.: Cambridge University Press, 1989.

Johnston, William. "Jūhasseiki Nihon no igaku ni okeru kagaku kakumei: ranpō no hatten no tame no shisōteki na zentei." *Nihon igaku zasshi* 27, no. 1 (1981): 6–20.

———. *The Modern Epidemic*. Cambridge, Mass.: Harvard University, Council on East Asian Studies, 1995.

Kadokawa Nihon chimei daijiten hensan iinkai, ed. *Nihon chimei daijiten*. 49 vols. Tokyo: Kadokawa, 1978–90.

Kaempfer, Engelbert. *Kaempfer's Japan: Tokugawa Culture Observed*. Translated by Beatrice Bodart-Bailey. Honolulu: University of Hawai'i Press, 1999.

Kanai Kōsaku. "Fukuda Kōsai no rangaku no michi to Agatsuma rangaku." *Gunma bunka* 203 (1985): 29–46.

———. "Rangaku to waga Nakanojōmachi." In *Nakanojōmachi shi*, ed. Nakanojōmachi shi hensan iinkai, pp. 1104–58. Nakanojōmachi, 1976.

———. *Takahashi Keisaku nikki*. Nakanojōmachi: Takahashi Keisaku nikki kankōkai, 1995.

———. "Takano Chōei monka Nakanojōmachi Mochizuki Shunsai no hizō monjo o haiken shite." *Gunma bunka* 247 (1996): 19–32.

———. *Takano Chōei to Agatsuma*. Nakanojōmachi: Kanai Kōsaku, 1992.

Kanai Kōsaku, ed. *Yanagida Teizō no Tenpō kiji*. Gunma: Jōmō shinbunsha, 1980.

Karasawa Sadaichi. *Agatsuma shichō*. Shichō shiriizu, vol. 9. Maebashi: Miyama bunko, 1998.

Kato, Shuichi. *A History of Japanese Literature*, vol. 2. Translated by Don Sanderson. Tokyo: Kodansha International, 1983.

Katsu Kokichi. *Musui's Story*. Translated by Teruko Craig. Tucson: University of Arizona Press, 1995.

Keene, Donald. *The Japanese Discovery of Europe, 1720–1830*. Stanford: Stanford University Press, 1969.

Kikuchi Isao. *Kinsei no kikin*. Tokyo: Yoshikawa kōbunkan, 1997.

Kiple, Kenneth F., ed. *The Cambridge World History of Human Disease*. Cambridge, Eng.: Cambridge University Press, 1993.

Klegon, Douglas. "The Sociology of Professions an Emerging Perspective." *Sociology of Work and Professions* 5, no. 3 (1978): 259–83.

Kodansha, ed. *Kodansha Encyclopedia of Japan*. 8 vols. Tokyo: Kodansha, 1983.

Koike Iichi. *Zusetsu Nihon no 'i' no rekishi*. Tokyo: Daikūsha, 1993.

Koike Zenkichi. *Edo jidai no Nakanojōmachi-machizukuri: jinkō, nōgyō*. 1963.

Kokushi daijiten henshū iinkai, ed. *Kokushi daijiten*. 14 vols. Tokyo: Yoshikawa kōbunkan, 1979–93.

Konta Yōzō. *Edo no hon'yasan*. Tokyo: NHK Books, 1977.

Kornicki, Peter. *The Book in Japan*. Leiden: Brill, 1998.

Koschmann, Victor. *The Mito Ideology*. Berkeley: University of California Press, 1987.

Kōseisho Imukyoku, ed. *Isei hyakunenshi*. Tokyo: Gyōsei, 1976.

Kure Shūzō, ed. *Shiiboruto Edo sanpu kikō*. Tokyo: Yūshōdō, 1966.

Kuriyama, Shigehisa. "Between Mind and Eye: Japanese Anatomy in the Eighteenth Century." In *Paths to Asian Medical Knowledge*, ed. Charles Leslie and Allan Young, pp. 21–43. Berkeley: University of California Press, 1992.

Kuriyama Shigehisa and Yamada Keiji, eds. *Rekishi no naka no yamai to igaku*. Kyoto: Kokusai Nihon bunka kenkyū sentā, 1997.

Lock, Margaret M. *East Asian Medicine in Urban Japan: Comparative Studies of Health Systems and Medical Care*. Berkeley: University of California Press, 1980.

Makino Tomitarō. *Shin Nihon shokubutsu zukan*. Tokyo: Hokuryūkan, 1962.

Maruyama Kiyoyasu. *Gunma no ishi*. Maebashi: Gunma ken ishi kai, 1958.

Matsuoka Hideo. "Kikin to sabetsu." In *Edo jidai no kikin*, ed. Kodama Kōta, Hayashiya Tatsusaburō, and Harada Tomohiko, pp. 131–34. Tokyo: Yūzankaku, 1982.

Mitani Hiroshi. "Rekishi no hōtei." *Nihon rekishi* 600, May (1998): 140–44.

Miyachi Masato. *Bakumatsu ishinki no bunka to jōhō*. Tokyo: Rekishigaku sōsho, 1994.

Miyashita, Saburo. "A Bibliography of the Dutch Medical Books Translated into Japanese." *Archives internationales d'histoire des sciences* 25 (1975): 8–72.

Moriya, Katsuhisa. "Urban Networks and Information Networks." In *Tokugawa Japan*, ed. Chie Nakane and Shinzaburo Oishi, pp. 97–123. Tokyo: University of Tokyo Press, 1990.

Morris, Ivan. *The Nobility of Failure*. New York: Holt, Rinehart and Winston, 1975.

Morris-Suzuki, Tessa. "Sericulture and the Origins of Japanese Industrialization." *Technology and Culture* 33, no. 1 (1992): 101–21.

———. *The Technological Transformation of Japan*. Cambridge, Eng.: Cambridge University Press, 1994.

Murakami Nao. "Kikin to daikan." In *Edo jidai no kikin*, ed. Kodama Kōta, Hayashiya Tatsusaburō, and Harada Tomohiko, pp. 134–36. Tokyo: Yūzankaku, 1982.

Najita, Tetsuo. "History and Nature in Eighteenth-Century Tokugawa Thought." In *The Cambridge History of Japan*, vol. 4, *Early Modern Japan*, ed. J. W. Hall, pp. 596–659. Cambridge, Eng.: Cambridge University Press, 1991.

Nakajima Yōichirō. *Byōki Nihonshi*. Tokyo: Yūzankaku shuppan, 1995.

———. *Kikin Nihonshi*. Tokyo: Yūzankaku, 1976.

Nakamura, Ellen Gardner. "A Portrait of Takano Chōei." *International Christian University Asian Cultural Studies* 24 (March 1998): 19–29.

Nakane, Chie, and Shinzaburo Oishi, eds. *Tokugawa Japan*. Tokyo: University of Tokyo Press, 1990.

Nakanojōmachishi hensan iinkai, ed. *Nakanojōmachishi shiryōhen*. Nakanojōmachi: Nakanojōmachi yakuba, 1983.

Nakayama, Shigeru. "Ways of Thinking of Japanese Physicians." Paper presented at the International Symposia on the Comparative History of Medicine—East and West, Shizuoka, Japan, 1976–77, pp. 3–19.

Nichiran gakkai, ed. *Yōgaku kankei kenkyū bunken yōran*. Tokyo: Nichigai Associates, 1984.

———. *Yōgakushi jiten*. Tokyo: Yūshōdō shuppan, 1984.

Numata Jirō. "Studies of the History of Yōgaku: A Bibliographical Essay." *Acta Asiatica* 42 (1982): 75–101.

———. *Yōgaku*. Tokyo: Yoshikawa kōbunkan, 1989.

Ōba Hideaki. *Hana no otoko Shiiboruto*. Tokyo: Bungei shunjū, 2001.

Ogawa Teizō. *Igaku no rekishi*. Chūō shinsho 39. Tokyo: Chūō kōronsha, 1964.

Ōishi Manabu. *Yoshimune to Kyōhō no kaikaku*. Tokyo: Tōkyōdō shuppan, 1995.

Ono Sanataka. *Edo no machiisha*. Tokyo: Shinchōsha, 1997.

Ōtsuki Fumihiko. "Takano Chōei gyōjō itsuwa." In *Fukken Zassan*, pp. 386–98. Tokyo: Kōbundō shoten, 1902.

Otsuka, Yasuo. "Chinese Traditional Medicine in Japan." In *Asian Medical Systems: A Comparative Study*, ed. Charles Leslie, pp. 322–40. Berkeley: University of California Press, 1976.

Ozaki, Norman Takeshi. "Conceptual Changes in Japanese Medicine During the Tokugawa Period." PhD diss., University of California, 1979.

Pearl, J. L. "The Role of Personal Correspondence in the Exchange of Scientific Information in Early Modern France." *Renaissance and Reformation* 8, no. 2 (1984): 106–13.

Peterson, M. J. *The Medical Profession in Mid-Victorian London*. Berkeley: University of California Press, 1978.

Porkert, Manfred. *Theoretical Foundations of Chinese Medicine*. Cambridge, Mass.: MIT Press, 1980.

Porter, Dorothy, and Roy Porter. *Patient's Progress*. Oxford: Polity Press, 1989.

Pratt, Edward. *Japan's Protoindustrial Elite*. Cambridge, Mass.: Harvard University Asia Center, 1999.

Riley, James C. *The Eighteenth-Century Campaign to Avoid Disease*. Basingstoke, Eng.: Macmillan, 1987.

Robertson, Jennifer. "Sexy Rice: Plant Gender, Farm Manuals, and Grass-Roots Nativism." *Monumenta Nipponica* 39, no. 3 (1984): 233–60.

Rosenberg, Charles E. "The Therapeutic Revolution: Medicine, Meaning, and Social Change in Nineteenth-Century America." *Perspectives in Biology and Medicine* 20, no. 4 (1977): 485–506.

Rubinger, Richard. *Private Academies of Tokugawa Japan*. Princeton: Princeton University Press, 1982.

Sansom, George. *The Western World and Japan*. London: Cresset, 1950.

Satō Shōsuke. *Takano Chōei*. Iwanami shinsho, shin akaban 512. Tokyo: Iwanami shoten, 1997.

———. *Watanabe Kazan*. Tokyo: Yoshikawa kōbunkan, 1986.

———. *Yōgakushi kenkyū josetsu*. Tokyo: Iwanami shoten, 1964.

———. *Yōgakushi no kenkyū*. Tokyo: Chūō kōronsha, 1980.

———. *Yōgakushi ronkō*. Kyoto: Shibunkaku shuppan, 1993.

Satō Shōsuke, ed. *Watanabe Kazan, Takano Chōei*. Nihon no meicho 25. Tokyo: Chūō kōronsha, 1972.

Screech, Timon. *The Western Scientific Gaze and Popular Imagery in Later Edo Japan: The Lens Within the Heart*. Cambridge, Eng.: Cambridge University Press, 1996.

Shils, Edward. "Center and Periphery." In *The Constitution of Society*, ed. Edward Shils, pp. 93–109. Chicago: University of Chicago Press, 1982.

Shinmura Taku. *Shussan to seishokukan no rekishi*. Tokyo: Hōsei daigaku shuppan kyoku, 1997.

Shirasugi Etsuo. "Nihon ni okeru kyūkōsho no seiritsu to sono engen." In *Higashi Ajia no honzō to hakubutsugaku no sekai*, ed. Yamada Keiji, pp. 138–73. Kyoto: Shibunkaku shuppan, 1995.

———. "Senki to Edo jidai no hitobito no shintai keiken." In *Rekishi no naka no yamai to igaku*, ed. Kuriyama Shigehisa and Yamada Keiji, pp. 63–92. Kyoto: Kokusai Nihon bunka kenkyu sentā, 1997.

Simmonds, N. W., ed. *Evolution of Crop Plants*. London: Longman, 1976.

Sippel, Patricia. "Aoki Konyō (1698–1769) and the Beginnings of *Rangaku*." *Japanese Studies in the History of Science* 11 (1972): 127–62.

Smith, F. Porter. *Chinese Materia Medica*. 2nd rev. ed. Taipei: Ku T'ing Book House, 1969.

Smith, Thomas. *The Agrarian Origins of Modern Japan*. Stanford: Stanford University Press, 1959.

Sōda Hajime. *Zusetsu Nihon iryō bunkashi.* Kyoto: Shibunkaku, 1989.

Steele, M. William, and John G. Caiger. "On Ignorant Whalers and Japan's 'Shell and Repel' Edict of 1825." *International Journal of Maritime History* 5, no. 2 (1993): 31–56.

Steger, Brigitte. "From Impurity to Hygiene: The Role of Midwives in the Modernisation of Japan." *Japan Forum* 6, no. 2 (1994): 175–87.

Sugimoto, Masayoshi, and David Swain. *Science and Culture in Traditional Japan A.D. 600–1854.* Cambridge, Mass.: MIT Press, 1978.

Sugiura Minpei. *Kazan to Chōei.* Tokyo: Daisan bunmeisha, 1977.

Sugiyama Shigeru. *Kusuri no shakaishi.* Tokyo: Kindaibungeisha, 1999.

Tabata Tsutomu. "Bakumatsu ni okeru ichi chihō ran'i no kiseki ni tsuite." *Chihōshi kenkyū* 191 (October 1984): 45–58.

Takano Chōei. "Wasuregatami." In *Nihon shisō taikei,* vol. 55, ed. Satō Shōsuke, pp. 171–84. Tokyo: Iwanami shoten, 1971.

Takano Chōei Kinenkan, ed. *Takano Chōei no tegami.* Mizusawa: Takano Chōei kinenkan, 1993.

Takano Chōei zenshū kankō kai, ed. *Takano Chōei zenshū.* 2nd ed. 6 vols. Tokyo: Daiichi shobō, 1978.

Takano Chōun. *Takano Chōei den.* 2nd ed. Tokyo: Iwanami shoten, 1943.

Takayanagi Kaneyoshi. *Edo jidai hinin no seikatsu.* Tokyo: Yūzankaku shuppan, 1981.

Taketa Katsuzō. *Furo to yu no koborebanashi.* Tokyo: Muramatsu shokan, 1977.

Takeuchi Makoto. "Shomin bunka no naka no Edo." In *Bunka no taishūka.* Nihon no kinsei 14, ed. Takeuchi Makoto, pp. 7–54. Tokyo: Chūō kōronsha, 1993.

Tanaka Yūko. *Edo no sōzōryoku.* Tokyo: Chikuma shobō, 1986.

Tanida Etsuji and Koike Mitsue. *Nihon fukushokushi.* Tokyo: Kōseikan, 1989.

Tasaki Tetsurō. *Chihō chishikijin no keisei.* Tokyo: Meicho shuppan, 1990.

———. "Yōgaku no denpan, fukyū." In *Bakumatsu no yōgaku,* ed. Nakayama Shigeru, pp. 51–65. Kyoto: Minerva shobō, 1984.

———. *Zaison no rangaku.* Tokyo: Meicho shuppan, 1985.

Tasaki Tetsurō, ed. *Zaison rangaku no tenkai.* Kyoto: Shibunkaku, 1992.

Tatsukawa Shōji. *Edo yamai no sōshi.* Tokyo: Chikuma shobō, 1998.

Toby, Ronald. *State and Diplomacy in Early Modern Japan.* Princeton: Princeton University Press, 1984.

Totman, Conrad. *Early Modern Japan.* Berkeley: University of California Press, 1993.

———. "Tokugawa Peasants: Win, Lose, or Draw." *Monumenta Nipponica* 41, no. 4 (1986): 457–76.

Tsukamoto Manabu. *Tokai to inaka.* Tokyo: Heibonsha, 1991.

———. "Toshi bunka to no kōryū." In *Mura no seikatsu bunka*. Nihon no kinsei 8, ed. Tsukamoto Manabu, pp. 333–82. Tokyo: Chūō kōronsha, 1992.

Uesugi Mitsuhiko. "Tenpō no kikin to bakuhan taisei no hōkai." In *Edo jidai no kikin*, ed. Kodama Kōta, Hayashiya Tatsusaburō, and Harada Tomohiko, pp. 105–15. Tokyo: Yūzankaku, 1982.

Vande Walle, W. F., and Kazuhiko Kasaya, eds. *Dodonaeus in Japan: Translation and the Scientific Mind in the Tokugawa Period*. Leuven and Kyoto: Leuven University Press and International Research Center for Japanese Studies, 2001.

Vaporis, Constantine. *Breaking Barriers*. Cambridge, Mass.: Harvard University, Council on East Asian Studies, 1994.

Waddington, Ivan. "General Practitioners and Consultants in Early Nineteenth Century England: The Sociology of an Intra-Professional Conflict." In *Health Care and Popular Medicine in Nineteenth Century England*, ed. John Woodward and David Richards, pp. 164–88. London: Croom Helm, 1977.

Wakabayashi, Bob Tadashi. *Anti-Foreignism and Western Learning in Early Modern Japan*. Cambridge, Mass.: Harvard University, Council on East Asian Studies, 1986.

Walker, Brett. "The Early Modern Japanese State and Ainu Vaccinations: Redefining the Body Politic, 1799–1868." *Past and Present* 163 (1999): 121–60.

Walter, John, and Roger Schofield, eds. *Famine, Disease and the Social Order in Early Modern Society*. Cambridge, Eng.: Cambridge University Press, 1989.

Walthall, Anne. "The Family Ideology of the Rural Entrepreneurs in Nineteenth Century Japan." *Journal of Social History* 23, no. 3 (1990): 463–84.

———. "The Lifecycle of Farm Women." In *Recreating Japanese Women, 1600–1945*, ed. Gail Lee Bernstein, pp. 42–70. Berkeley: University of California Press, 1991.

———. "Village Networks Sōdai and the Sale of Edo Nightsoil." *Monumenta Nipponica* 43, no. 3 (1988): 279–303.

Watanabe Kazan. "Gaikoku jijōsho." In *Nihon shisō taikei*, vol. 55, ed. Sato Shōsuke. Tokyo: Iwanami shoten, 1971.

Watanabe Shin'ichirō. *Edo no onnatachi no yuami*. Tokyo: Shinchōsha, 1996.

White, James. "State Growth and Popular Protest in Tokugawa Japan." *Journal of Japanese Studies* 14, no. 1 (1988): 1–25.

Willis, Evan. *Medical Dominance*. Sydney: George Allen and Unwin, 1983.

Wittermans, Elizabeth P., and John Z. Bowers, eds. *Doctor on Desima: Selected Chapters from Jhr J. L. C. Pompe van Meerdervoort's "Vijf Jaren in Japan."* Tokyo: Sophia University, 1970.

Yamada Keiji, ed. *Mono no imeeji honzō to hakubutsugaku e no shōtai.* Tokyo: Asahi shinbunsha, 1994.

Yanai Kenji, ed. *Nagasaki Dejima no shokubunka.* Nagasaki: Shinwa bunko, 1993.

Yoshioka Shin. *Edo no kigusuriya.* Tokyo: Seiabō, 1994.

Index

Harvard East Asian Monographs
(* out-of-print)

Harvard East Asian Monographs

Harvard East Asian Monographs

Harvard East Asian Monographs

Harvard East Asian Monographs

Harvard East Asian Monographs